COLOUR GUIDE

CW00395219

Periodontology

Peter Heasman BDS, MDS, FDS RCPS, DRD RCS, PhD
Senior Lecturer and Honorary Consultant, Department of Restorative
Dentistry, The Dental School, University of Newcastle upon Tyne, UK

Philip Preshaw BDS, FDS RCS (Edin)
Research Fellow, Department of Restorative Dentistry, The Dental School,
University of Newcastle upon Tyne, UK

David Smith BDS, DRD RCS (Edin), FDS RCS (Edin), FDS RCS (Eng)
Consultant and Postgraduate Dental Dean, Department of Restorative
Dentistry, The Dental School, University of Newcastle upon Tyne, UK

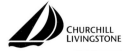

CHURCHILL
LIVINGSTONE

NEW YORK EDINBURGH LONDON MADRID MELBOURNE
SAN FRANCISCO TOKYO 1997

CHURCHILL LIVINGSTONE
Medical Division of Pearson Professional Limited

Distributed in the United States of America by
Churchill Livingstone Inc., 650 Avenue of the
Americas, New York, N.Y. 10011, and by
associated companies, branches and
representatives throughout the world.

© Pearson Professional Limited 1997
except figures listed in acknowledgements

The rights of Peter Heasman, Philip Preshaw and
David Smith to be identified as authors of this
work have been asserted by them in accordance
with the Copyright, Designs and Patents Act 1988.

First published 1997

ISBN 0 443 05705 2

British Library Cataloguing in Publication Data
A catalogue record for this book is available from
the British Library.

**Library of Congress Cataloging in Publication
Data**
A catalog record for this book is available from
the Library of Congress.

Medical knowledge is constantly
changing. As new information
becomes available, changes in
treatment, procedures, equipment
and the use of drugs become
necessary. The authors and the
publishers have, as far as it is
possible, taken care to ensure
that the information given in this
text is accurate and up to date.
However, readers are strongly
advised to confirm that the
information, especially with
regard to drug usage, complies
with current legislation and
standards of practice.

The
publisher's
policy is to use
**paper manufactured
from sustainable forests**

Produced by Longman Asia
Limited, Hong Kong
SWTC/01

Acknowledgements

The authors wish to acknowledge the invaluable skills and expertise of Brian Hill and Janet Howarth of the Department of Dental Photography at Newcastle Dental Hospital. We are also indebted to Claire Grainger for the preparation and editing of numerous drafts of the manuscript.

Some of the periodontal conditions and many of the syndromes covered in this book are extremely rare and we have only been able to illustrate these with the help and generosity of our professional colleagues: Professor Hubert Newman (Eastman Dental Institute), Dr Iain Chapple (Birmingham Dental School), Professor Robin Seymour, Professor Jim Soames, Dr Anita Nolan, Mr Andrew Shaw, Dr June Nunn, Dr Ian Macgregor, Dr Richard Welbury, Dr Mark Thomason, Mr Nigel Carter, Mr Finbarr Allen, Mr David Jacobs, Mr Eoin Smart and Mr David Murray (Newcastle Dental School and Hospital).

We also gratefully acknowledge permission for use of the following illustrations:
Figures 67, 112, 117 and 157 from Heasman PA, Millett DT 1996 The Periodontium and Orthodontics in Health and Disease, Oxford University Press.
Figures 81 and 107 from Seymour RA, Heasman PA 1992 Drugs Diseases and the Periodontium, Oxford University Press.
Figures 124, 125 and 126 from Heasman PA, McLeod I, Smith DG 1994 Factitious Gingival Ulceration: a presenting sign of Munchausen's Syndrome, Journal of Periodontology Vol 65
Figures 39, 40, 43, 44, 46, 47, 49, 50, 52 and 53 from Heasman PA, Smith DG 1988 The Role of Anatomy in the Initiation and Spread of Periodontal Disease, Dental Update Vols 1 & 2

Contents

Mature periodontal tissues

The diagnostic skills required to identify periodontal diseases are based upon a sound knowledge of normal periodontal anatomy.

Clinical features

Gingiva is pink, firm in texture and extends from the free gingival margin to the mucogingival line (Fig. 1). Interdental papillae are pyramidal in shape and occupy the interdental space beneath the tooth contact points. Gingiva is keratinised and stippling is frequently present. The gingiva is comprised of:

- ◊free gingiva, which is the most coronal band of unattached tissue sometimes demarcated by the free gingival groove.
- ◊attached gingiva, which is firmly bound to underlying cementum and alveolar bone. It extends apically from the free gingival groove to the mucogingival junction. The width of attached gingiva varies considerably throughout the mouth.

The depth of the gingival sulcus ranges from 0.5–3.0 mm. A serum exudate, gingival crevicular fluid, flows from the gingival capillary network into the sulcus at a rate of approximately 20 μl/h. The mucogingival line is often indistinct. It defines the junction between the keratinised attached gingiva and the oral mucosa. Oral lining mucosa is non-keratinised and thus redder than the adjacent gingiva. The tissues can be distinguished by staining with Schiller iodine solution: keratinised gingiva is stained orange and non-keratinised mucosa purple-blue (Fig. 2).

Radiographic features

The crest of the interdental alveolar bone is well defined and lies approximately 0.5–1.5 mm apical to the cemento-enamel junction (CEJ) (Fig. 3). ▶

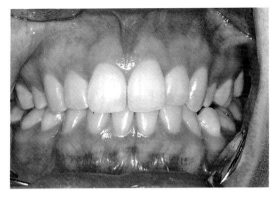

Fig. 1 Healthy gingiva.

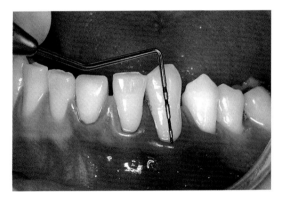

Fig. 2 Gingiva and oral mucosa stained with iodine.

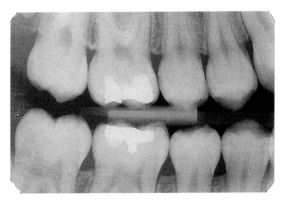

Fig. 3 Healthy alveolar bone.

Histology

Epithelial components (Figs 4, 5):

- Junctional epithelium cells are non-keratinised and attached to the tooth surface by a basal lamina and hemidesmosomes.
- Sulcular epithelium is non-keratinised and lines the gingival crevice.
- Oral epithelium is keratinised from the free gingival margin to the mucogingival line.

Gingival connective tissue   core contains ground substance; blood vessels and lymphatics; nerves; fibroblasts and bundles of gingival collagen fibres: dentogingival, alveologingival, circular, trans-septal (Figs 4, 5). The combined epithelial and gingival fibre attachment to the tooth surface is the *biologic width*.

Periodontal connective tissues   comprise alveolar bone; periodontal ligament principal and oxytalan (Figs 6, 7) fibres, cells, ground substance, nerves, blood vessels and lymphatics; cementum.

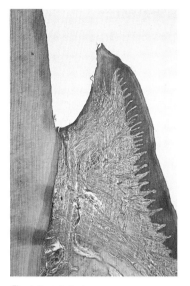

Fig. 4 Buccal gingiva.

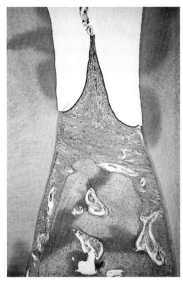

Fig. 5 Interproximal gingiva.

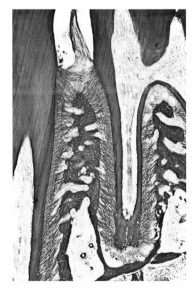

Fig. 6 Periodontal ligament principal fibres.

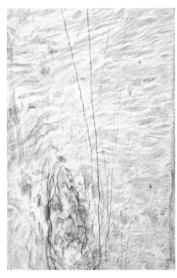

Fig. 7 Fine black staining oxytalan fibres.

Periodontal tissues in children

Clinical features

Gingiva may appear red and inflamed. Compared to mature tissue there is:
- thinner epithelium which is less keratinised
- greater vascularity of connective tissues
- less variation in the width of attached gingiva.

During tooth eruption gingival sulcus depths may exceed 5 mm and gingival margins will be at different levels on adjacent teeth. Following tooth eruption a persistent hyperaemia can lead to swollen and rounded interproximal papillae (Fig. 8).

Radiographic features

In primary dentition the radiographic distance between the CEJ and the alveolar crest is 0–2 mm. Greater variation (0–4 mm) is observed at sites adjacent to erupting permanent teeth and exfoliating primary teeth (Fig. 9). The periodontal membrane space is wider in children due to thinner cementum, immature alveolar bone and a more vascular periodontal ligament.

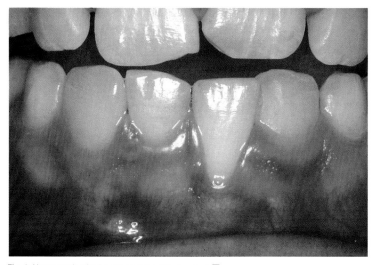

Fig. 8 Hyperaemic gingiva around recently erupted /1̄.

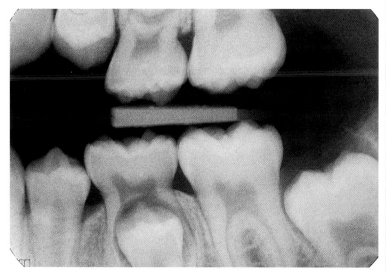

Fig. 9 Alveolar crest morphology—mixed dentition.

Dental plaque

An accumulation of bacteria and intercellular matrix which adheres to the surfaces of teeth and other oral structures in the absence of effective oral hygiene.

Classification

Supragingival plaque is located on the clinical crowns of teeth whereas subgingival plaque is found within the gingival sulcus or periodontal pocket.

Supragingival plaque

Clinical features

A soft, yellow-white layer on the tooth surface which accumulates primarily at the free gingival margin (Fig. 10). It can be detected by the naked eye or by running a probe around the gingival margin. Disclosing solutions greatly facilitate the detection of plaque (Fig. 11) and are useful for demonstrating supragingival plaque to patients.

Microbiology

Bacterial colonisation of the tooth surface begins within a few hours of tooth cleaning. Gram-positive cocci and rods constitute the majority of the microorganisms, with *Streptococci* and *Actinomyces* species predominating. After 48 hours the numbers of all types of bacteria increase though their relative proportions alter and Gram-negative cocci and rods become more prevalent. After about 4 days fusobacteria and filamentous bacteria proliferate. Spirochaetes are present after approximately one week. The growth conditions in thick, mature plaque favour a complex flora comprising predominantly anaerobic Gram-negative species. ➡

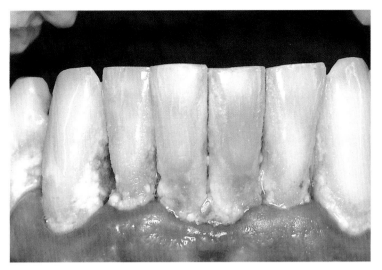

Fig. 10 Supragingival plaque.

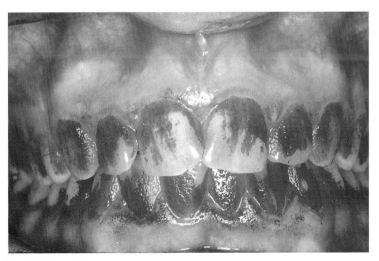

Fig. 11 Disclosed plaque.

Subgingival plaque

Clinical features

Develops from the downgrowth of supragingival plaque into the gingival sulcus or periodontal pocket. Subgingival plaque cannot be seen directly unless the overlying gingiva is retracted (Fig. 12) or the plaque is removed from within the gingival sulcus with a periodontal probe.

Microbiology

Unique environmental conditions exist in the gingival sulcus which favour colonisation and growth of anaerobic bacteria. There is protection from cleansing mechanisms within the oral cavity, and gingival crevicular fluid supplies a ready flow of nutrients.

In a shallow gingival sulcus the mixed bacterial flora comprises principally *Streptococci* and *Actinomyces* species. Gram-negative rods include *Fusobacteria* and *Campylobacter* species. At periodontally diseased sites Gram-negative rods and motile species, including spirochaetes, account for the vast majority of the plaque bacteria, resulting in a complex aggregation of densely packed anaerobic organisms (Fig. 13).

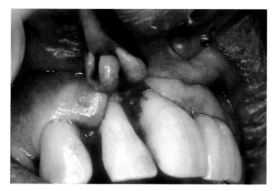

Fig. 12 Subgingival plaque and calculus on distal surface of 1̲/.

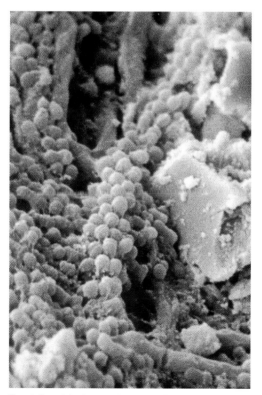

Fig. 13 Scanning electron micrograph of plaque bacteria.

Dental calculus

A hard, mineralised substance which forms on the surfaces of teeth and other solid structures in the oral cavity following the prolonged accumulation of dental plaque. Approximately 90% of adults exhibit calculus (UK Adult Dental Health Survey, 1988).

Composition

Dental plaque is mineralised by calcium and phosphate ions from saliva. Inorganic calcium phosphate crystals develop within the plaque matrix and enlarge until the plaque is mineralised. Calculus crystals grow in contact with enamel, dentine and cementum, gaining mechanical retention in tooth surface irregularities. The outer surface of calculus remains covered by a layer of unmineralised plaque.

Classification

Supragingival calculus is located on the clinical crowns of teeth whereas subgingival calculus is present within the gingival sulcus or periodontal pocket.

Supragingival calculus

Clinical features

Yellow-white calcified deposits primarily located at, or just above, the gingival margins. Stain brown with tobacco and certain foods or drinks (Fig. 14) (p. 15). Frequently found opposite the duct openings of major salivary glands, on the lingual aspect of mandibular incisors and canines (Fig. 14) and the buccal surfaces of maxillary molars (Fig. 15). Deposits can grow to a considerable size, forming on occlusal surfaces of unopposed teeth and on surfaces of fixed or removable prostheses (Fig. 16). ➡

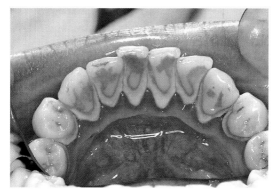

Fig. 14 Supragingival calculus and tobacco staining.

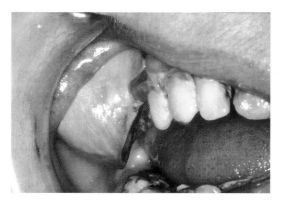

Fig. 15 Gross supragingival calculus opposite opening of parotid duct.

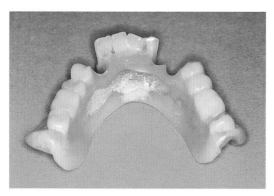

Fig. 16 Calculus on polished surface of denture.

Subgingival calculus

Dark brown-green deposits located beneath the gingival margin, adhering firmly to the root surface. Found particularly at interproximal sites.

If the gingival margin is dried, the dark colour of subgingival calculus may be seen through the marginal soft tissues. A fine calculus probe is used to detect deeper subgingival calculus, and interproximal deposits may be seen on radiographs (Fig. 17).

Direct vision of subgingival calculus facilitates its removal, and is achieved:

- using a gentle stream of air to reflect the gingival margin
- following gingival recession (Fig. 18)
- during periodontal surgery.

'Subgingival calculus' is occasionally seen on dentures when it forms in narrow grooves, such as those at the tooth–acrylic interface (Fig. 19).

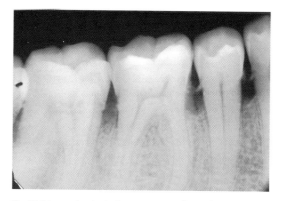

Fig. 17 Interproximal calculus seen on a radiograph.

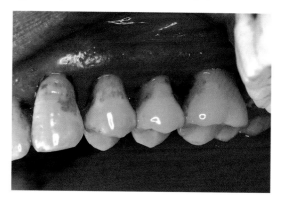

Fig. 18 Interproximal subgingival calculus exposed following gingival recession.

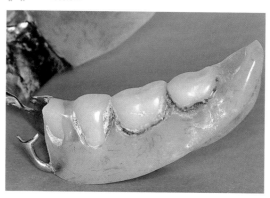

Fig. 19 Calculus in 'gingival crevice' of denture.

Extrinsic stains

Tobacco smoke
Tobacco smoking results in a dark brown stain on the tooth surface, particularly affecting the palatal/lingual aspects of anterior teeth (Fig. 14) (p. 12). These sites are exposed to exhaled smoke and are often neglected by the smoker during tooth cleaning.

Dietary factors
Tea, coffee and other pigmented foods and drinks—particularly when consumed frequently—also stain plaque and calculus.

Chlorhexidine gluconate (CHX)
An antimicrobial active against a broad spectrum of bacteria. Available as a mouthrinse (0.2% or 0.12% w/v) for the control of plaque and gingivitis. Prolonged use causes brown staining of the hard and soft tissues of the oral cavity (Fig. 20). The mechanism of staining is uncertain and various theories have been proposed:

- CHX reacts with dietary ketones and aldehydes to form insoluble coloured compounds.
- CHX denatures pellicle proteins resulting in pigmented products.
- CHX catalyses the polymerisation of carbohydrates and amino acids to produce brown pigmented melanoids.

Chromogenic bacteria
When dental plaque contains chromogenic bacteria it has a characteristic unsightly green-brown hue (Fig. 21). Easily removed by scaling and polishing.

Habitual chewing
Prolonged and frequent usage of chewing tobacco and betel nut results in a striking pattern of extrinsic black staining (Fig. 22).

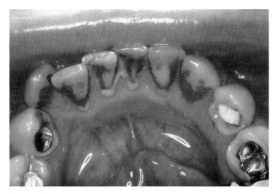

Fig. 20 Chlorhexidine stain.

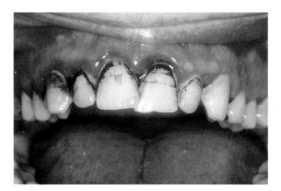

Fig. 21 Chromogenic green stain.

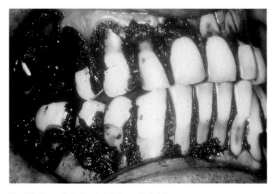

Fig. 22 Gross betel nut debris and staining.

Chronic gingivitis

Definition

A plaque-induced, inflammatory lesion of the gingiva.

Incidence

26% of 5-year-olds, 62% of 9-year-olds and 52% of 15-year-olds have gingivitis (Children's Dental Health Survey, UK, 1993). About 80% of adults have some evidence of bleeding gums and 69% have shallow pockets (Adult Dental Health Survey, UK, 1988).

Clinical features

Gingiva are red, shiny, swollen and soft, or spongy in texture. Sulcus depths increase (false pockets) as a result of the tissue swelling due to inflammatory oedema. Bleeding occurs after gentle probing. The interdental papillae and marginal gingiva are initially involved before inflammation spreads to the attached gingiva (Fig. 23).

Aetiology

Accumulation of dental plaque in the gingival sulcus initiates the development of an inflammatory lesion (subclinical) which, after 10–20 days, is detected clinically as an established chronic gingivitis.

Pathology

Developing lesion is manifested by intense vasculitis with a protein-rich serum exudate, degeneration of perivascular collagen, deposition of fibrin and a predominantly neutrophil/monocyte infiltrate (Fig. 24). After a few days the cellular infiltrate becomes lymphocytic but with some plasma cells at the periphery. These developing stages of gingival inflammation have been observed in the experimental gingivitis model. How they relate to development of spontaneous, plaque-induced gingivitis is unclear.

Established gingivitis (Fig. 25) demonstrates all the changes of 'developing' lesions but with greater numbers of plasma cells. Sulcular epithelium degenerates into 'pocket' epithelium which proliferates laterally into the gingival connective tissue. ▶

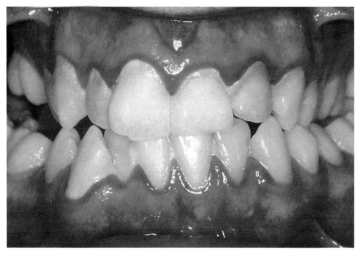

Fig. 23 Marginal gingivitis.

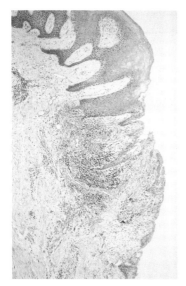

Fig. 24 Early inflammatory infiltrate.

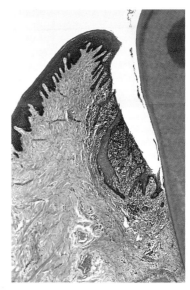

Fig. 25 Histopathology of established gingivitis.

Gingivitis in children is dominated by lymphocytes although smaller numbers of neutrophils and plasma cells are present. This suggests stability or quiescence rather than a progressing lesion.

Sequela | *Untreated,* an established lesion remains stable for an indefinite period of time or progresses to an advanced, destructive lesion—chronic periodontitis (p. 23).

Treatment | Instruction in toothbrushing and use of interdental cleaning aids. Supragingival scaling, elimination of plaque retentive factors (p. 31), subgingival scaling and polishing.

Pregnancy gingivitis

Clinical features | A generalised, marginal, oedematous gingivitis (Fig. 26). The extent of gingival enlargement is variable but an increase in gingival bleeding is a common complaint. The severity of the gingivitis tends to increase from the second to the eighth month of pregnancy. There is often some resolution during the final trimester and after parturition. A local gingival overgrowth—pregnancy epulis—may result from chronic irritation or mild trauma to the soft tissues (p. 85).

Aetiology | An increase in circulating levels of oestrogen, progesterone and their metabolites aggravates a pre-existing or subclinical gingivitis. The hormones and their metabolites effect an increase in gingival vasculature and the permeability of the capillary network. A similar increase in the severity of an established gingivitis may also be seen at, or around, puberty (Fig. 27) and with long-term use of oral contraceptives.

Treatment | A preventive regimen is preferred whenever possible. Otherwise conventional treatment approach including oral hygiene instruction and scaling.

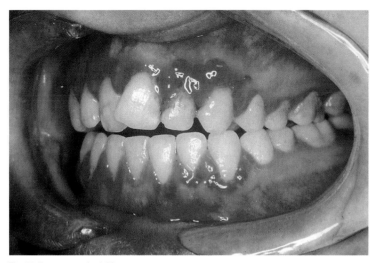

Fig. 26 Pregnancy gingivitis.

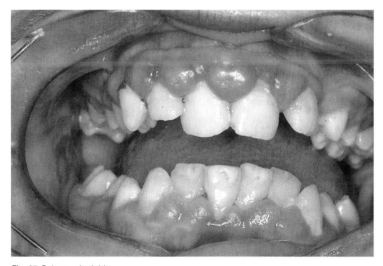

Fig. 27 Puberty gingivitis.

Plasma cell gingivitis

A contact hypersensitivity reaction most frequently attributed to cinnamon flavoured chewing gum. Cinnamon, mint and herbal flavoured toothpastes are also implicated.

Clinical features

Gingivae are fiery red in appearance (Fig. 28) with varying degrees of swelling. The lesion extends to involve the entire width of attached gingiva. The reaction may affect other areas such as the tongue, palate and cheeks. Lips can be dry and desquamative with an angular cheilitis. The principal symptom is extreme soreness of the affected areas.

Pathology

Atrophic epithelium and a massive infiltrate of plasma cells in the connective tissues.

Treatment

Identification and withdrawal of the causative allergen. If toothbrushing is painful during the acute stage, chlorhexidine mouthrinse can be given for chemical plaque control.

Desquamative gingivitis

Not a discrete clinical entity. A term used to describe a gingival manifestation common to plasma cell gingivitis and mucocutaneous disorders: benign mucous membrane pemphigoid (p. 127); lichen planus (p. 125); pemphigus vulgaris (p. 127). The fiery-red, desquamative lesions affect the entire width of keratinised gingiva and may be localised or generalised throughout the mouth (Fig. 29).

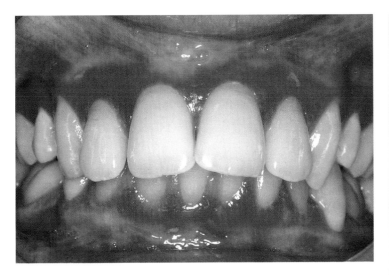

Fig. 28 Plasma cell gingivitis.

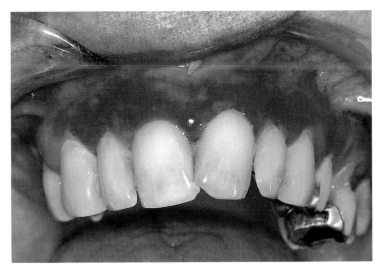

Fig. 29 Desquamative gingivitis in benign mucous membrane pemphigoid.

Chronic adult periodontitis

Periodontitis is bacterially-induced inflammation of the periodontium.

Incidence

Only 5% of dentate adults are completely free of any signs of periodontitis. 69% of adults have early signs of the disease and 10% have at least one deep periodontal pocket of 6 mm or greater (Fig. 30) (Adult Dental Health Survey, UK, 1988).

Clinical features

Pocketing   *True* periodontal pockets result from apical migration of the junctional epithelium (JE) following loss of connective tissue attachment to the root surface. A degree of *false* pocketing (p. 17) resulting from gingival oedema or fibrosis is usually present. In *suprabony* pockets the JE remains entirely coronal to the alveolar crest whereas in *infrabony* pockets the JE extends apically beyond the alveolar crest.

Different types and designs of periodontal probe are available for measuring probing pocket depth, the distance from the free gingival margin to the position of the probe tip, which is assumed to be located at the base of the pocket at the level of the JE. Accuracy of measurement of pocket depths is dependent upon:
- design and diameter of the probe tip (sharp, blunt, ball-ended)
- probing force (maximum recommended 25 g)
- degree of inflammation in the soft tissues
- position, angulation and orientation of the probe
- presence of calculus
- root morphology
- restricted access and/or visibility.

Bleeding on probing (Fig. 31)   occurs at inflamed sites where thin and ulcerated junctional and pocket epithelia are not resistant to penetration by the probe tip. ➡

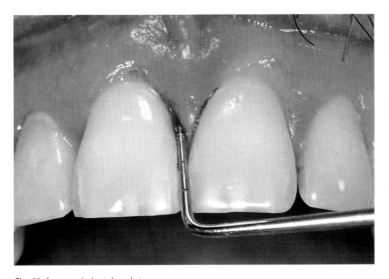

Fig. 30 6 mm periodontal pocket.

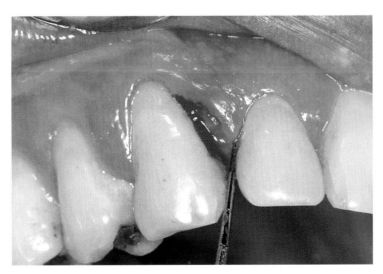

Fig. 31 Bleeding following probing of pocket.

Alveolar bone resorption occurs concurrently with attachment loss and pocket formation. Two distinct patterns of bone destruction are recognised radiographically. *Horizontal* bone loss occurs when the entire width of interdental bone is resorbed evenly (Fig. 32). *Vertical* bone defects are produced when the interdental bone adjacent to the root surface is more rapidly resorbed, leaving an angular, uneven morphology (Fig. 33). Frequently, both patterns of bone resorption are seen in the same patient.

Tooth mobility is either:
- *physiological*, which allows slight movements of a tooth within the socket to accommodate masticatory forces, without injury to the tooth or its supporting tissues.
- *pathological*, with increased or increasing mobility as a result of connective tissue attachment loss. Pathological mobility is dependent on the quantity of remaining bony support, the degree of inflammation in the periodontal ligament and gingiva and the magnitude of occlusal or any jiggling forces (p. 103) which may be acting upon the teeth. A reduction in mobility follows treatment and resolution of inflammation.

Tooth mobility is measured by displacing the tooth with a rigid dental instrument and a moderate force (Fig. 34):
- Grade I: horizontal mobility <1 mm
- Grade II: horizontal mobility ≥1 mm
- Grade III: horizontal mobility >2 mm and/or vertical mobility. ➡

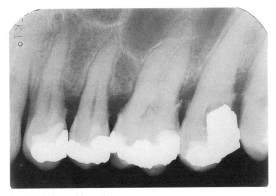

Fig. 32 Horizontal bone loss.

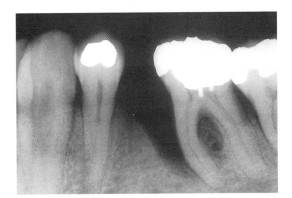

Fig. 33 Vertical bone loss.

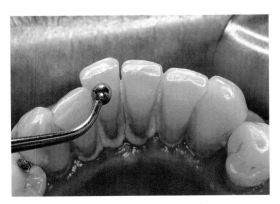

Fig. 34 Testing tooth mobility.

Migration of teeth may occur following attachment loss or gingival overgrowth. It frequently affects maxillary incisors which drift labially, resulting in increased overjet and diastemata (Fig. 35). Such teeth also have a tendency to over-erupt.

Gingival recession may be localised or generalised. *Localised* recession is associated with factors such as toothbrush trauma, high frenal attachment, factitious injury, bony dehiscence or thin alveolar bone (p. 91).

  Generalised recession occurs when the gingival margin migrates apically as a result of ongoing periodontal disease or following resolution of gingival inflammation and oedema as a consequence of treatment (p. 92).

Furcation lesions arise when attachment loss occurs vertically and horizontally between the roots of multi-rooted teeth. Lesions are detected using:
- direct visualisation
- a furcation probe (Fig. 36)
- radiographic examination (Fig. 37).

A probe is required to classify furcations:
- Class I: horizontal attachment loss $<\frac{1}{3}$ tooth width
- Class II: horizontal attachment loss $>\frac{1}{3}$ tooth width (but not complete horizontal attachment loss)
- Class III: complete horizontal attachment loss ('through and through' lesion). ➡

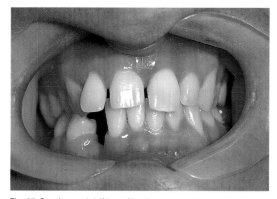

Fig. 35 Spacing and drifting of teeth.

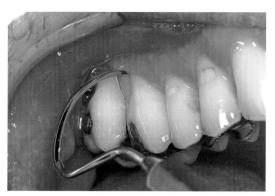

Fig. 36 Probing a grade II furcation.

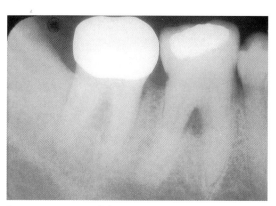

Fig. 37 Furcation lesion $\overline{6}$/.

Histopathology	The transition from established gingivitis to periodontitis constitutes the development of an advanced lesion (Fig. 38). These changes are preceded by a shift in lymphocyte populations from the T cell predominated early lesion to one in which B lymphocytes and plasma cells predominate. The pocket epithelium is very thin, ulcerated, and permeable to bacterial products, inflammatory mediators and defence cells. Inflammatory changes subjacent to junctional epithelium (JE) extend laterally and apically. Connective tissue fibres apical to the JE are degraded by collagenases. This is followed by proliferation of JE in an apical direction.

Exposed cementum adsorbs bacterial products and becomes soft and necrotic. The prospect of repair is minimal unless the necrotic tissue is removed during root planing. Osteoclast bone resorption is driven by plaque and host-derived mediators such as bacterial enzymes, prostaglandins, interleukins and tumour necrosis factor.

Treatment

- *Oral hygiene instruction*: systematic toothbrushing technique and interproximal cleaning aids (dental floss, mini-interdental brushes, interspace brushes)
- *Scaling and root planing* to remove subgingival plaque, calculus and necrotic cementum
- *Re-evaluation* to assess the response to treatment, reinforce oral hygiene instruction and provide further instrumentation if necessary.

Sites refractory to conventional therapy may be considered for:

- locally delivered antimicrobials
- periodontal surgery.

Furcation treatment depends upon the severity of the lesions. Options include:

- scaling and root planing
- surgical flap elevation gaining direct access for instrumentation
- furcationplasty
- guided tissue regeneration
- tunnel preparation
- root resection
- extraction.

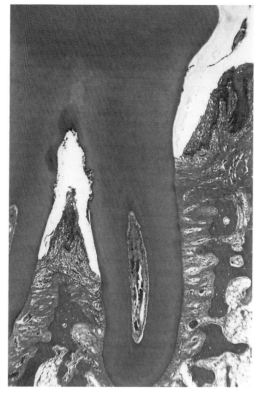

Fig. 38 Histopathology of chronic periodontitis.

Local anatomical factors associated with the teeth and the supporting tissues may imitate, initiate, or predispose to periodontal disease.

Tooth anatomy

Crown shape and length

Bulbous clinical crowns predispose to accumulation of plaque below the line of maximum contour. Plaque and calculus also form in, and are difficult to remove from, a prominent cemento-enamel junction. Long clinical crowns give the impression of gingival recession when cementoenamel junctions (CEJ) are more apical than those on adjacent teeth (Fig. 39). Small, conical or 'peg shaped' crowns with no contact point(s) allow the adjacent marginal gingiva to proliferate leading to deepening of the gingival sulcus and loss of contour of the interdental papillae (Fig. 40).

Cervical enamel projections (CEP)

Projections of the CEJ into, and/or through, the furca of molars (Fig. 41). Notches of the adjacent alveolar bone crest are sometimes associated with CEPs. The periodontal attachment to the enamel of a CEP is epithelial, making these sites susceptible to periodontal disease progression.

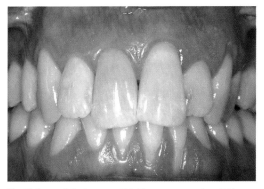

Fig. 39 Long clinical crowns 1|1. Note true recession /̄1̄2̄.

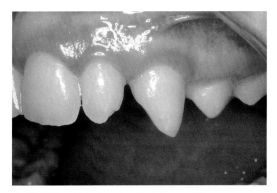

Fig. 40 Flattened interdental papilla between /23.

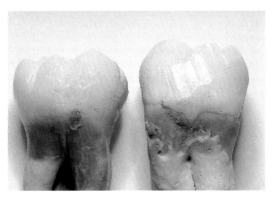

Fig. 41 Cervical enamel projections.

Root morphology

An appreciation of the variation and complexity of root anatomy is crucial to understanding how periodontal disease can be more advanced around certain teeth. Plaque and calculus accumulate readily in pronounced concavities and deep grooves on root surfaces. Palatoradicular grooves, which are present on about 50% of maxillary lateral incisors (Fig. 42), frequently extend to the apical third of the root (Fig. 43), and can appear as an extra root canal on periapical radiographs (Fig. 44). Local, deep and tortuous infrabony defects are frequently associated with such grooves, requiring surgical exploration. Deeper grooves are often proximal to, or may communicate with, root canals so odontoplasty must be undertaken with extreme care.

Supplemental roots, narrow furcal entrances, and concavities on the mesial and distal roots of molars can all severely restrict access for root instrumentation (Fig. 45).

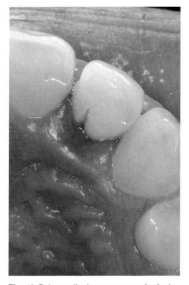

Fig. 42 Palatoradicular groove at gingival margin.

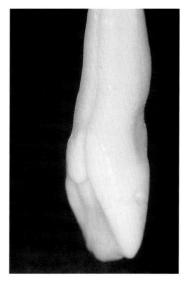

Fig. 43 Palatoradicular groove on extracted tooth.

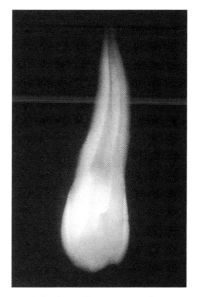

Fig. 44 Radiographic appearance of a palatoradicular groove.

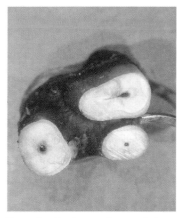

Fig. 45 Restricted access for root planing between molar roots.

Furcation ridges

Pronounced ridges of cementum that run in a mesio-distal direction across the furca of multi-rooted teeth (Fig. 46). They may also be situated across the buccal or lingual openings of furca and so limit access for instrumentation or self-performed plaque control. When accessible they can be removed using tapered or torpedo diamond burs (odontoplasty).

Enamel pearls

Droplets of enamel found on root surfaces. Pearls are isolated or linked to the CEJ by a ridge of enamel. Pearls have no connective tissue attachment and are formed when small sheets of Hertwig's root sheath maintain their contact with dentine during root formation. If present in a periodontal pocket a pearl may be mistaken for subgingival calculus and can be an obstacle to effective root planing (Fig. 47).

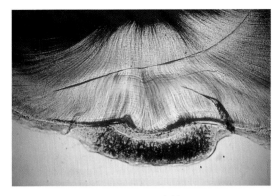

Fig. 46 Intermediate furcation cemental ridge.

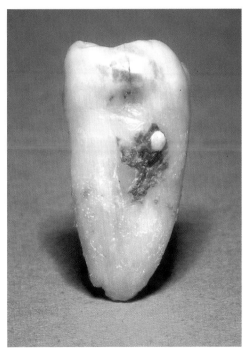

Fig. 47 Enamel pearl and subgingival calculus.

Tooth–arch relationships

Crowded dentition

Imbricated or overlapping teeth result in increased plaque accumulation in the absence of effective self-performed cleaning. Gingivitis develops, although there is no evidence to suggest that overcrowding is a risk factor for destructive periodontitis. Localised crowding may also lead to displacement of a single tooth from the arch, thus creating a stagnation area (Fig. 48). The gingiva tends to increase in thickness as it proliferates into the gap from which the tooth is displaced. This 'excess' tissue further compromises the practice of effective oral hygiene.

Contact points

In areas of crowding, contact points may be lost or 'converted' into long contact lines between teeth. Tight contacts make interdental cleaning virtually impossible because of the restricted access for floss, woodpoints and interdental brushes (Fig. 49). ➡

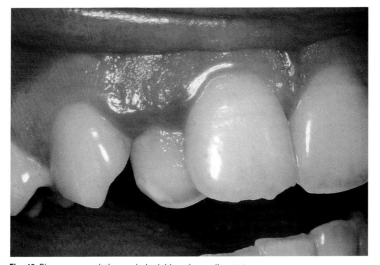

Fig. 48 Plaque accumulation and gingivitis at instanding 2/.

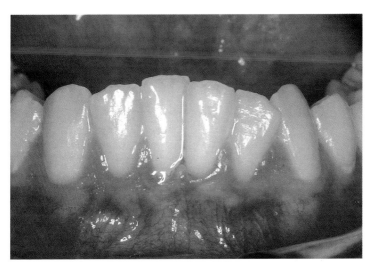

Fig. 49 Tight contacts between incisors.

Single standing teeth

Teeth adjacent to an edentulous span have a tendency to drift, tilt, tip or overerupt. Frictional forces of food shedding mechanisms are lost and unopposed mesial and distal surfaces in particular become stagnation sites for plaque and debris (Fig. 50).

'Stacked' molars

The proximity of roots of 'stacked' maxillary molars allows for only a very thin plate of interproximal bone. The restricted access for cleaning between 'stacked' molars makes these sites susceptible to plaque accumulation and the very thin interproximal alveolar bone is rapidly resorbed (Fig. 51).

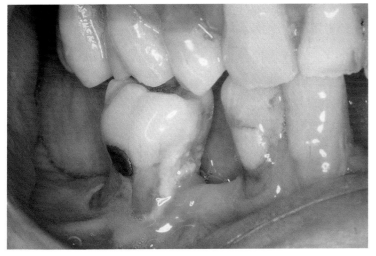

Fig. 50 Plaque on mesial surface of free-standing tooth.

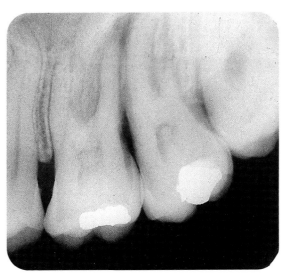

Fig. 51 'Stacked' maxillary molars.

Alveolar bone

Microanatomy

The pattern of bone resorption in periodontal disease is determined by the width and density of the alveolar crest. Generally, the buccal and lingual cortical plates are more likely to resist the spread of inflammation than cancellous bone at interproximal sites. Interdental foramina are numerous between premolars and molars and transmit many small vessels between the bone and the gingiva (Fig. 52). Preferential resorption of cancellous alveolar crest leads to the formation of 'crater' or 'saucer' defects between and around posterior teeth.

Macroanatomy

Dehiscences and fenestrations are gaps or 'windows' in alveolar bone which are frequently associated with prominent or irregular roots (Fig. 53). In the absence of periodontal disease, teeth with such associated defects appear to be at no greater risk of gingival recession. The rate of progression of established recession may, however, increase at a dehiscence or fenestration.

Local excrescences of bone are developmental in nature and appear as hard swellings on the attached gingiva. These exostoses may be single, bilateral (for example torus mandibularis/palatinus), or multiple when they appear on the buccal surface of the maxilla just below the mucobuccal fold (Fig. 54). The covering epithelium is thin and at risk from trauma which may result from incorrect or overzealous toothbrushing.

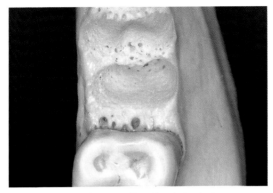

Fig. 52 Foramina at the crest of interdental alveolar bone.

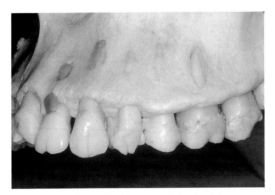

Fig. 53 Fenestrations and dehiscences of alveolar plates.

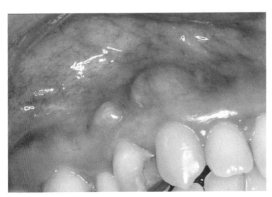

Fig. 54 Bony exostoses of the maxilla.

Soft tissues

Gingival sulcus

Partially or recently erupted teeth with immature marginal gingiva demonstrate a degree of false pocketing which remains for 3 to 4 years until the junctional epithelium migrates apical to the CEJ. False 'pockets' are also common on the distal sites of third (or last standing) molars where the bulky tissues of the retromolar pads or the tuberosities abut the teeth (Fig. 55).

Frenal attachments

A 'high' labial or buccal frenum has traditionally been implicated as a risk factor for localised gingival recession. The most significant problem associated with a prominent frenum, however, is the restriction of access for toothbrushing as a result of the reduction in sulcus depth (Fig. 56). Surgical separation (frenotomy) or excision (frenectomy) is indicated if plaque control is a persistent problem despite local oral hygiene measures. ➡

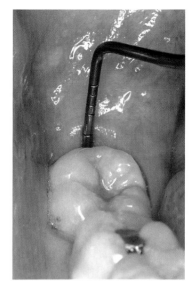

Fig. 55 False pockets distal to third molar.

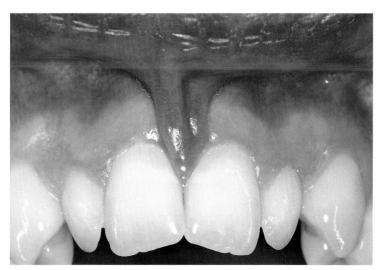

Fig. 56 Broad attachment of maxillary midline frenum.

Incompetent lips

Caused by weak muscle tone and increased overjet of maxillary incisors (Fig. 57). The lack of lip seal leads to mouth breathing, usually in the absence of nasal obstruction.

Clinical features

A marginal, oedematous and erythematous gingivitis may be localised to the anterior maxillary segment. The amount of gingival enlargement is variable (Fig. 58). The gingivitis is plaque-induced and aggravated by drying of plaque on teeth, drying of the gingiva and the lack of functional self-cleansing mechanisms.

Treatment

- Instructions in oral hygiene.
- Use of barrier paste (Vaseline).
- Orthodontic opinion regarding correction of incisor relationship.

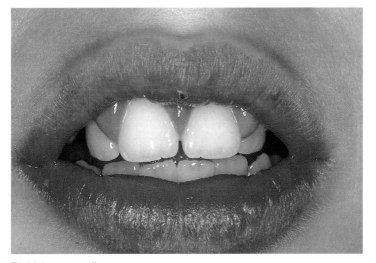

Fig. 57 Incompetent lips.

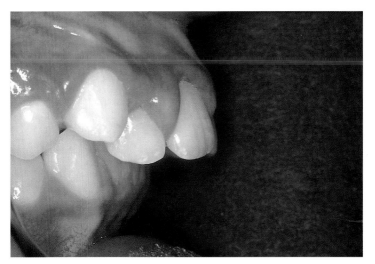

Fig. 58 Increased overjet, gingivitis and gingival enlargement.

Overhanging restorations

Result from poor technique when restoring teeth. Amalgam and composite 'flash' overhangs occur frequently at interproximal sites and are avoided by ensuring that matrix bands or strips are closely adapted to the tooth surface. Overhangs render interproximal cleaning impossible and result in plaque-induced inflammation (Fig. 59), loss of attachment and alveolar bone destruction (Fig. 60).

Treatment
- Where access permits, remove overhang with a fine diamond bur or a flat diamond stone in a horizontally reciprocating handpiece (Eva ® handpiece).
- Replace restoration if necessary.
- Oral hygiene instruction (OHI) interproximal cleaning, scaling, root planing.

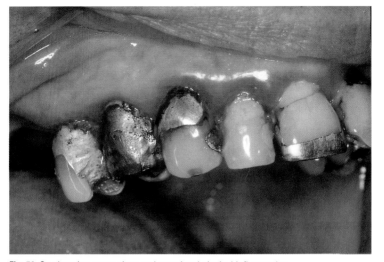

Fig. 59 Overhanging restorations and associated gingival inflammation.

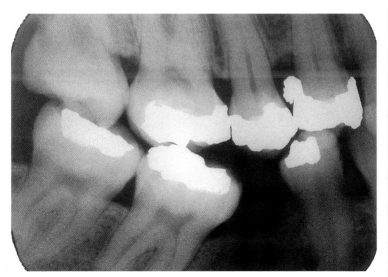

Fig. 60 Amalgam overhang and bone destruction 4̲ / distal.

Defective crown margins

Supragingival crown margins are easy to clean but may compromise appearance. Subgingival margins are generally indicated at aesthetically important sites but care must be taken not to compromise the biologic width of attachment (p. 3). Crown margins should not 'interrupt' the normal contour of the tooth surface.

Classification

A *positive* crown margin extends beyond the intended margin of the prepared tooth (Fig. 61). A *negative* defect finishes short of the margins of the preparation.

Clinical features

Defective margins inevitably result in plaque accumulation even if the overall standard of oral hygiene is high. Gingival tissues are erythematous, oedematous and bleed on probing (Fig. 62).

Treatment

- At try-in, reject crowns with defective margins and take new impressions.
- Small positive defects may be corrected with fine diamond burs and polishing stones.
- Replace the defective crown.

Bridge pontics

Bridge pontics must be carefully designed to facilitate cleaning and minimise plaque accumulation. This is achieved by ensuring the pontics are clear of the gingival tissues. A compromise between aesthetics and cleansibility is usually necessary. Pontics should have smooth surfaces, be convex in all directions and have minimal, light contact on the buccal surface of the edentulous ridge. This allows for self-performed cleaning with superfloss and is aesthetically pleasing.

Clinical features

Pontics which impinge on the soft tissues increase plaque accumulation and inflammation (Fig. 63). Aesthetics are compromised as a result of poor soft tissue appearance.

Treatment

- OHI (superfloss), scaling.
- Recontour the pontic.
- Replace bridge.

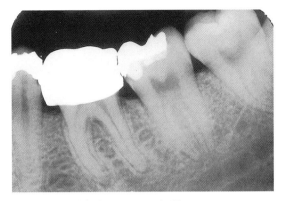

Fig. 61 Positive defective crown margin $\overline{6}$.

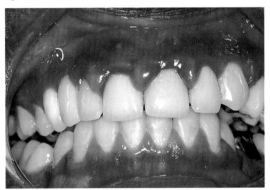

Fig. 62 Gingival inflammation associated with defective margins of crowned maxillary teeth.

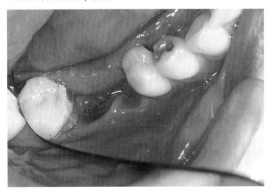

Fig. 63 Inflamed soft tissue revealed after removing defective bridge pontics.

Partial dentures

Removable prostheses encourage plaque accumulation in the absence of effective oral hygiene.

Clinical features

Acrylic dentures with interproximal collets (Fig. 64) ('gum strippers') cause plaque-induced inflammation, destructive periodontitis and recession of the gingival tissues (Fig. 65). Framework components and clasps of cobalt–chrome dentures positioned too close to the gingival margin aggravate plaque-induced inflammation, and occasionally cause direct trauma.

Prevention

- Utilise tooth support in preference to mucosal support.
- Ensure adequate clearance of the gingival tissues by saddles, major and minor connectors and clasps.
- Avoid interproximal collets.
- Simplify denture design where possible.

Treatment

- Replace poorly designed dentures.
- OHI and denture hygiene (clean denture with a toothbrush and water; leave denture out at night).

Orthodontic appliances

Fixed and removable appliances encourage plaque accumulation. Fixed appliances require considerable effort to keep brackets, bands, wires, elastics and tooth surfaces plaque free. Removable appliances can be taken from the mouth to be cleaned and allow toothbrushing.

Clinical features

Plaque-induced gingivitis in the region of the appliance (Fig. 66).

Prevention

- Appliances should not be provided for patients who are unable to practise good oral hygiene.
- Ensure adequate clearance of the gingival tissues.
- Simplify appliance design.

Treatment

OHI; mini-interdental and interproximal brushes, superfloss.

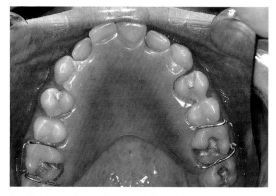

Fig. 64 Interproximal collets on maxillary denture.

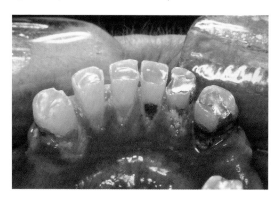

Fig. 65 Chronic periodontitis aggravated by an all-acrylic lower partial denture.

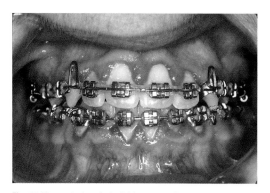

Fig. 66 Plaque-induced gingivitis around fixed orthodontic appliance.

Basic periodontal examination[1] (BPE)

A convenient, easily performed screening system to identify the periodontal status and treatment needs of individual patients. The World Health Organisation periodontal probe (Fig. 67) is designed specifically for this purpose and has a 0.5 mm diameter ball-end and a coloured band at 3.5–5.5 mm from the tip. For screening, the dentition is divided into sextants:

RIGHT	7–4	3–3	4–7	**LEFT**
	7–4	3–3	4–7	

Each sextant must contain a minimum of two functioning teeth. A sextant with only one tooth is recorded as 'missing' and the score for that tooth is included in the adjacent sextant. Pocket depth is measured around every tooth in each sextant but only the *highest score* (deepest pocket) is recorded.

Score 0

Gingiva with no pockets or bleeding after probing (Fig. 68).

Treatment

None.

Score 1

No calculus and no overhanging margins of restorations. Bleeding occurs after probing. Coloured band remains completely visible (no pocket depths >3 mm) (Fig. 69).

Treatment

Oral hygiene instruction (OHI). ➡

---

[1] *Periodontology in general dental practice in the United Kingdom. A first policy statement.* 1992. British Society of Periodontology.

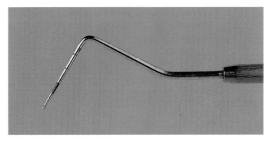

Fig. 67 World Health Organisation probe.

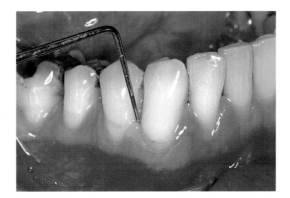

Fig. 68 BPE score 0.

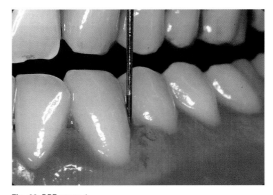

Fig. 69 BPE score 1.

Score 2	Calculus (supra- or sub-gingival) present and/or overhanging restorations. Bleeding occurs after probing. Coloured band remains completely visible (Fig. 70).
Treatment	OHI; scaling; correction of defective margins.
Score 3	Pocket depth of 4 or 5 mm. Coloured band of probe remains partly visible (Fig. 71).
Treatment	OHI; plaque and bleeding scores; scaling; correction of defective margins.
Score 4	Pocket depth of 6 mm or greater. Coloured band of probe completely disappears into pocket (Fig. 72).
Treatment	OHI; full periodontal assessment (plaque, bleeding and probing scores); radiographic examination; scaling and root planing; correction of defective margins; referral to a specialist may be appropriate.
Score*	Used to indicate furcation involvement or recession plus probing depth of 7 mm or more.
Treatment	As for Score 4.

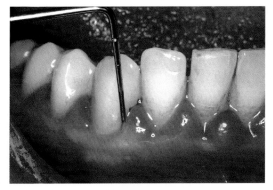

Fig. 70 BPE score 2.

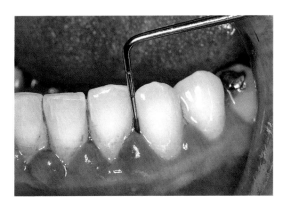

Fig. 71 BPE score 3.

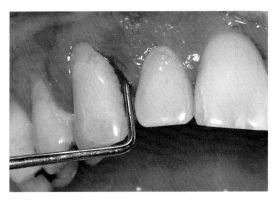

Fig. 72 BPE score 4.

Acute necrotising ulcerative gingivitis (ANUG)

An acute condition which has characteristic signs and symptoms and a tendency to recur.

Incidence

In Europe and the USA the incidence is 0.5–0.7% in the 16–30 age group. In African countries a more severe, aggressive form of ANUG is found in children as young as 1–2 years old.

Clinical features

'Punched out' ulcers covered with a yellow-grey pseudomembranous slough (Figs 73, 74). The tips of interdental papillae are first affected, but spread to the labial and lingual marginal gingiva can be rapid. ANUG is very painful and accompanied by a distinctive halitosis. A pre-existing, or longstanding chronic gingivitis is usually present. Fever and regional lymphadenopathy are associated only with severe cases.

Aetiology

A fusiform—spirochaetal complex is traditionally associated with ANUG (Fig. 75). Gram-negative anaerobic species are also implicated: *Porphyromonas gingivalis, Veillonella*, and *Selenomonas*.

Pathology

Ulceration of gingival epithelium with necrosis of subjacent connective tissues. Superficially, deposits of fibrin are intermeshed with large numbers of dead and dying cells: epithelial; neutrophils; bacteria. Deeper tissues demonstrate a dense infiltrate of neutrophils characteristic of non-specific inflammation. ➡

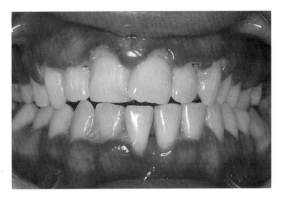

Fig. 73 ANUG.

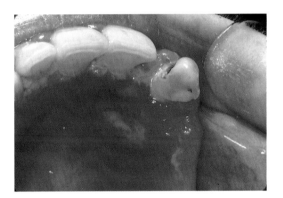

Fig. 74 Ulceration of palatal gingiva and mucosa.

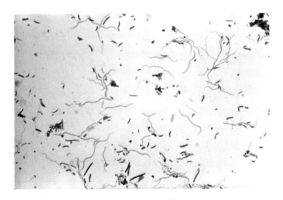

Fig. 75 Fuso-spirochaetal bacterial complex.

Risk factors	*Pre-existing gingivitis* confirms a poor standard of plaque control.
	Smoking favours the development of an anaerobic Gram-negative flora and depresses the chemotactic response of neutrophils.
	Mental stress, producing high plasma levels of hydrocorticosteroids, predisposes to ANUG and is a possible explanation for epidemics in college students and army personnel.
	Malnutrition and debilitation predispose to infection and severe ANUG in underdeveloped countries.
Differential diagnosis	Primary herpetic gingivostomatitis; HIV gingivitis.
Treatment	Reduce cigarette consumption. Oral hygiene instruction and ultrasonic scaling. If mechanical therapy is painful, or if fever and regional lymphadenopathy are present, then a 3-day course of systemic metronidazole, 200 mg t.d.s., is indicated. Oxygenating mouthrinses (hydrogen peroxide, sodium hydroxyperborate) cleanse necrotic tissues. Subgingival scaling and prophylaxis are essential to prevent recurrence.
Complications	Incomplete treatment leads inevitably to recurrence and loss of gingival contour (Fig. 76). A longstanding necrotising gingivitis may progress to a chronic necrotising (ulcerative) periodontitis (Fig. 77).

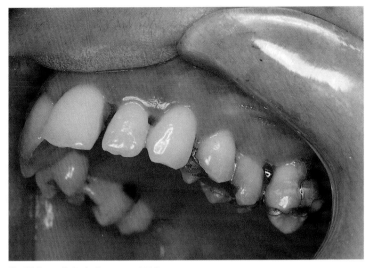

Fig. 76 Loss of gingival contour /123.

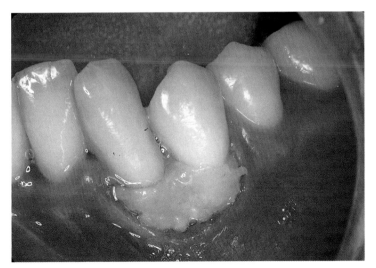

Fig. 77 Chronic necrotising ulcerative periodontitis with exposed bone.

Primary herpetic gingivostomatitis

Aetiology

An acute, common and highly infectious disease caused by Herpes simplex virus. Most adults have neutralising antibodies to the virus and circulating maternal antibodies provide immunity in the first 12 months. Transmission of the virus is predominantly by droplet infection and the incubation period is about 5–10 days.

Clinical features

Primary infection occurs most frequently in young children but can affect young adults.

Symptoms are fever, pyrexia, headaches, general malaise, dysphagia and regional lymphadenopathy.

Signs are an aggressive marginal gingivitis (Fig. 78) and formation of fluid-filled vesicles on the gingiva, tongue, palate and buccal mucosa. Vesicles burst after only a few hours to leave painful, yellow-grey ulcers with red, inflamed margins (Fig. 79). Ulcers heal without scarring after about 14 days.

Treatment

Mainly palliative. Bed rest, soft diet and maintain fluid intake. Paracetamol suspension for pyrexia. In severe cases give acyclovir, 200 mg, as a suspension to swallow, 5 times daily for 5 days. In young children, control plaque with chlorhexidine spray 2 or 3 times a day.

Complications

In immunocompromised patients the disease can be very severe and run a protracted course. Other complications—aseptic meningitis and encephalitis—are very rare.

Recurrent herpetic gingivostomatitis

Aetiology

Latent Herpes virus dormant in host's sensory ganglia is reactivated by exposure to sunlight, stress, nutritional deficiency, malaise, or systemic upset.

Clinical features

Attenuated presentation of the primary infection. Herpes labialis presents as a 'cold sore' at the mucocutaneous borders or commissures of the lips (Fig. 80).

Treatment

Cold sores managed with topical acyclovir cream (5%), 5 times a day, for 5–7 days.

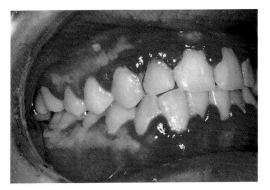

Fig. 78 Herpetic gingivostomatitis.

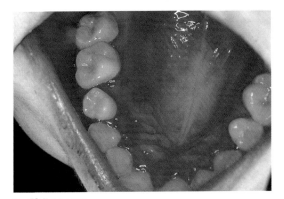

Fig. 79 Palatal lesions.

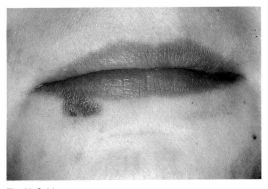

Fig. 80 Cold sore.

Acquired immune deficiency syndrome (AIDS)

Infection with human immunodeficiency virus (HIV) primarily targets the CD4 helper lymphocytes leading to a severe state of immunosuppression. Macrophages are also infected. Patients are susceptible to a range of opportunistic bacterial, viral, protozoal and fungal infections as well as neoplasms and neurological disturbances.

Clinical features

Common oral manifestations are generalised candidiasis and hairy leukoplakia. HIV infection is also associated with specific periodontal diseases.

HIV gingivitis (Fig. 81)
Characterised by a well-defined erythema of the marginal gingiva. The gingivitis may become more generalised and is resistant to conventional therapy.

HIV periodontitis (Figs 82, 83)
Rapidly progressing destruction of the gingiva with ulceration and cratering. Necrosis may be widespread, affecting soft and hard tissues, leading to sequestration of alveolar bone. The condition is extremely painful.

Microbiology

The microflora is typical of that associated with an advanced chronic or early onset periodontitis: *Porphyromonas gingivalis; Prevotella intermedius; Fusobacterium nucleatum; Eikenella corrodens; Campylobacter recta; Actinobacillus actinomycetemcomitans*. Fungal infection with *Candida albicans* is usual.

Pathogenesis

Suppression of cellular host response mechanisms effectively increases the virulence of the periodontopathogens. Neutrophil function is not compromised as these cells are primed to a level of hyperactivity, possibly by the chronic exposure to bacteria.

Treatment

Oral hygiene instruction, scaling and root planing. Chlorhexidine gluconate mouthrinse (0.2%, twice daily) and local irrigation with Betadine (1% povidone–iodine, up to 3 times daily) control the growth of plaque. Sodium perborate or hydrogen peroxide mouthwashes for oxygenation and superficial debridement of necrotic tissue.

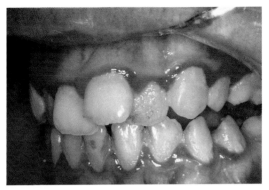

Fig. 81 HIV marginal gingivitis.

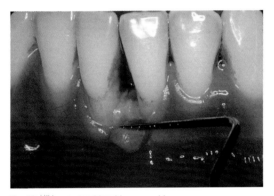

Fig. 82 HIV periodontitis with exposed bone.

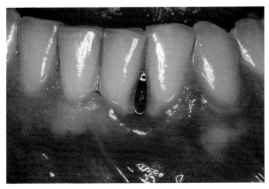

Fig. 83 HIV periodontitis with soft tissue craters.

Definition	An acute suppurative inflammatory lesion within the periodontal pocket or gingival sulcus.
Aetiology	Usually arises from: • an acute exacerbation of chronic periodontitis • trauma to the pocket epithelium (from instrumentation, toothbrush bristles, food impaction) • orthodontic movement of teeth through untreated, periodontally compromised tissues.
Clinical features	• Gingival erythema (Fig. 84) • Swelling of the overlying gingiva (Fig. 85) • Discharge of pus from the gingival margin (may be spontaneous) • Pain from the affected site made worse by biting • Unpleasant taste.
Diagnosis	• Tooth is tender to percussion • Acute pain on probing, with discharge of pus and blood • Vitality testing to distinguish from acute periapical periodontitis • Radiographs.
Treatment	• Incision if drainage cannot be achieved through pocket • Subgingival instrumentation and irrigation with chlorhexidine • Warm saline mouthrinses to encourage further drainage • Systemic antimicrobials; metronidazole 400 mg t.d.s. for 5 days is effective against anaerobes. Penicillins may also be prescribed • Re-evaluation to assess response to treatment and prognosis of the affected tooth.

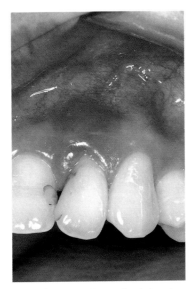

Fig. 84 Gingival erythema of periodontal abscess.

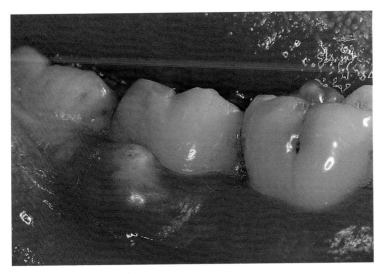

Fig. 85 Pointing periodontal abscess.

Definition

An inflammatory lesion originating in either the pulp or the periodontal ligament with the potential to spread from one site to the other via a number of pathways: apical foramina; lateral and furcation accessory root canals; exposed dentinal tubules; and root defects caused by caries, fractures, or perforations during operative procedures.

Classification

There are five types, based upon pathogenic interactions of pulpal–periodontal disease.

Primary endodontic lesions

Aetiology

Infection from a necrotic pulp drains into the periodontium to produce a periapical abscess. This remains localised, drains coronally through the periodontal membrane and gingival sulcus, or tracks through the alveolar bone to leave a swelling and a sinus opening in the attached gingiva (Fig. 86). There is no periodontal aetiology.

Clinical features

Persistent discomfort rather than frank pain. Negative response of tooth to vitality test. Periapical radiolucency on radiograph which may show evidence of spread coronally (Fig. 87). No loss of alveolar bone height on mesial and distal alveolar crest. Furcation bone loss between molar roots suggests spread of infection via accessory furcation canal.

Treatment

Root canal therapy.

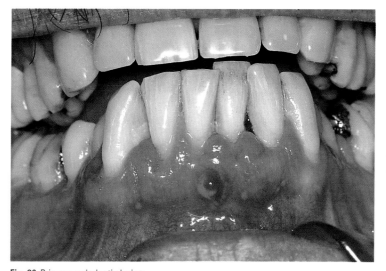

Fig. 86 Primary endodontic lesion.

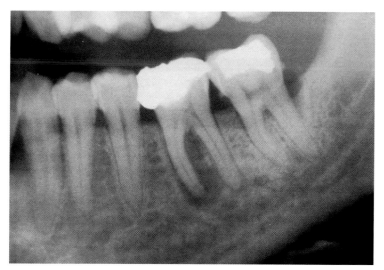

Fig. 87 Coronal spread of periapical infection.

Endodontic lesions with secondary periodontal involvement

Aetiology

Untreated or inadequately managed endodontic lesion which becomes a persistent source of infection to the marginal periodontium.

Clinical features

Similar to those of primary endodontic lesions. Gingival inflammation, increased probing pocket depth (Fig. 88), bleeding or pus on probing may be evident. Subgingival plaque and calculus are detected. Radiographs show periapical radiolucency and some resorption of crestal alveolar bone (Fig. 89).

Treatment

Root canal therapy or replacement of a previous, unsatisfactory root filling. Oral hygiene measures, scaling and prophylaxis. Extraction should be considered in the case of an extensive lesion.

Primary periodontal lesions (p. 65)

Aetiology

Periodontal infection which spreads to involve the periapical tissues. This may be associated with a local anatomical defect such as a radicular groove on a maxillary lateral incisor.

Clinical features

Localised, longstanding pain or discomfort. Positive response of tooth to vitality test. Gingivitis and localised deep pocketing with pus and bleeding following probing or application of pressure to the gingiva. Radiographs show localised bone resorption (Fig. 90) which can appear as horizontal, vertical, furcation and even 'apical' defects. Anatomical predisposing factors may occasionally be detected.

Treatment

Oral hygiene instruction, scaling and root planing. Surgical treatment to improve access for instrumentation or to eliminate anatomical factors. Consider use of locally-delivered antimicrobials if infection persists. Consider extraction in the case of an extensive lesion.

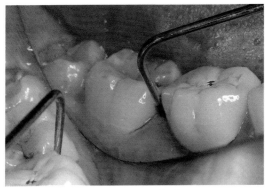

Fig. 88 Clinical probing of lesion on /6̄ distal.

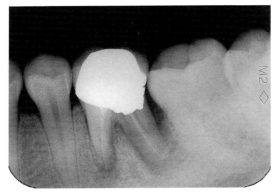

Fig. 89 Spread of periapical infection to involve marginal periodontium of /6̄ .

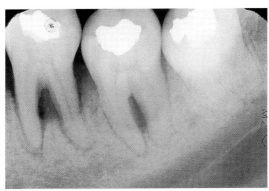

Fig. 90 Primary periodontal lesions /6̄7̄ .

Periodontal lesions with secondary endodontic involvement

Aetiology

Infection spreads from the periodontium to the pulp causing pulpitis and necrosis.

Clinical features

Similar to those of primary periodontal lesions but the tooth gives a negative response to vitality testing. The radiographic appearance may be identical to teeth with periodontal involvement only, although bone loss is generally more extensive (Fig. 91). Conversely, narrow, tortuous defects can be associated with grooves on the root surface.

Treatment

Root canal therapy. Oral hygiene instruction, scaling and root planing. Consider use of local antimicrobials if infection persists. Surgery to facilitate access to deeper pockets/anatomical defects or to undertake regenerative procedures. Consider extraction in the case of an extensive lesion.

True combined lesions

Aetiology

A periodontal infection 'coalesces' with a periapical lesion of pulpal origin. There are two distinct origins (Fig. 92).

Clinical features

Same as above. The remaining periodontal attachment is often minimal so tooth mobility is significant.

Treatment

As above, but for multi-rooted teeth consider root amputation, hemisection, or extraction. The prognosis is often very poor.

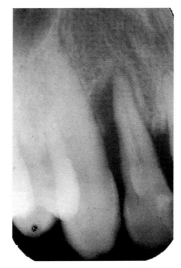

Fig. 91 Periodontal infection spread to involve apex of ⟍2⟋.

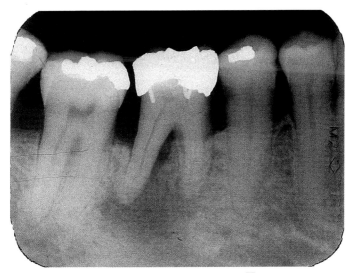

Fig. 92 Combined periodontal–endodontic lesion on distal root 6⟋.

Superficial staining

Caused by various foods and drinks, tobacco (smoking or chewing), and betel nut.

Racial pigmentation

Due to the production of melanin by melanocytes in the basal cell layer of the epithelium (Fig. 93).

Amalgam tattoo

A localised blue-black area of discolouration commonly affecting mandibular mucosa (Fig. 94). Results from the spillage of amalgam into the soft tissues during dental procedures (placement or removal of amalgam restorations, extraction of teeth containing amalgam restorations, apicectomies with amalgam retrograde root fillings). Typically asymptomatic, often an incidental finding.

Addison's disease

Adrenocortical insufficiency which usually results from bilateral tuberculosis of the adrenal glands or autoimmune adrenal failure. Brown or blue pigmentation of the skin, gingiva (Fig. 95) and oral mucosa may be the presenting sign and is due to increased secretion of adrenocorticotrophic hormone (ACTH) by the pituitary gland which is believed to have a melanocyte-stimulating action. Progressive or deepening pigmentation of recent onset should arouse suspicion of hypo-adrenocorticism.

Heavy metal salts

Extremely rare. Excessive or chronic exposure to mercury, lead, or bismuth results in precipitation of these metals as sulphides from crevicular fluid. Visible as a thin blue-black line of discolouration of the free gingival margin.

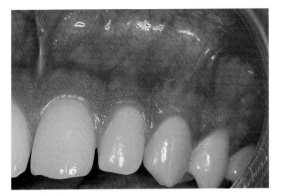

Fig. 93 Racial pigmentation.

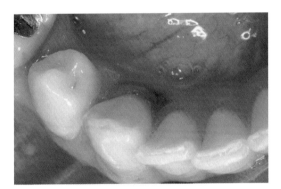

Fig. 94 Amalgam tattoo.

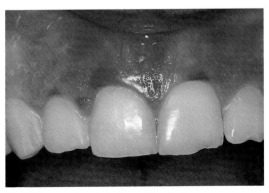

Fig. 95 Pigmentation of gingiva—Addison's disease.

12 / Gingival enlargement

Classification

Generalised gingival enlargement (Fig. 96)
Fibrous overgrowths:
- gingival fibromatosis
- chronic hyperplastic gingivitis
- drug associated gingival overgrowth.

Oedematous enlargement:
- hormonal gingivitis (p. 19).

Systemic diseases:
- acute leukaemia
- Crohn's disease
- orofacial granulomatosis
- sarcoidosis
- Wegener's granulomatosis.

Localised gingival enlargement (Fig. 97)
Hyperplastic lesions:
- epulides
  — fibrous
  — vascular
  — peripheral giant cell granuloma
- iatrogenic
  — denture induced
  — orthodontically induced

Cystic lesions
Neoplastic lesions (Ch. 19).

History

Gingival enlargement may occasionally be the first presenting sign of an underlying systemic disorder. A full medical history should always be taken, and clinicians must be alert for additional signs and symptoms to confirm the diagnosis. A systemic approach will reveal the medication history, haemorrhagic tendencies, abdominal and gastrointestinal upset, or any respiratory problems. Careful extra- and intra-oral examinations are necessary to determine the nature and extent of the lesion, additional signs, and predisposing or traumatic factors. Referral to a specialist centre for additional investigations may be appropriate.

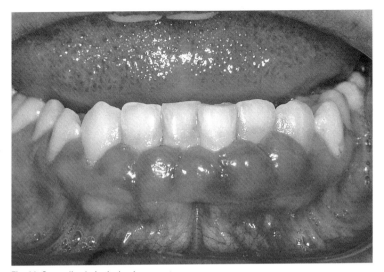

Fig. 96 Generalised gingival enlargement.

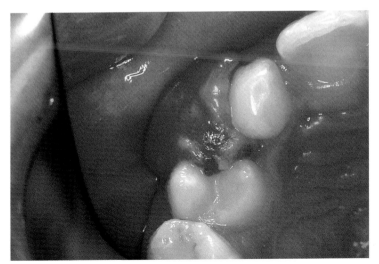

Fig. 97 Localised gingival enlargement.

Gingival fibromatosis

Uncommon condition with autosomal dominant inheritance pattern.

Clinical features

Generalised fibrous enlargement of the gingiva due to the accumulation of bundles of collagen fibres. Frequently associated with fibrous enlargement of the maxillary tuberosities (Fig. 98).

Treatment

Usually not required, unless access for cleaning is impaired or aesthetics are compromised. Tends to recur following surgical excision.

Chronic hyperplastic gingivitis

May occur following prolonged accumulation of dental plaque. Frequently associated with concomitant systemic medications (p. 79) though predisposing factors may not be identifiable.

Clinical features

Firm, pink gingival enlargement, particularly at interdental sites. May partially cover the crowns of teeth, resulting in aesthetic problems and cleaning difficulties (Fig. 99).

Treatment

Oral hygiene instruction; scaling; gingivectomy.

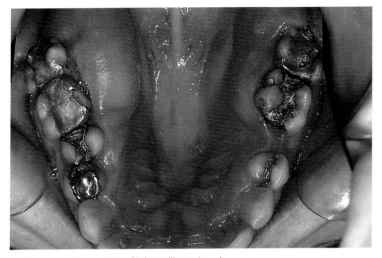

Fig. 98 Gingival fibromatosis of left maxillary tuberosity.

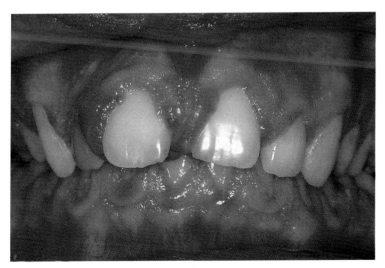

Fig. 99 Chronic hyperplastic gingivitis.

Drug associated gingival overgrowth

Phenytoin, cyclosporin and the calcium-channel blockers (notably nifedipine) are all associated with gingival overgrowth.

Incidence

Varies between the different drugs, affecting approximately 50% of patients medicated with phenytoin and 30% and 20% for cyclosporin and nifedipine respectively. Prevalence is increased in children and adolescents.

Clinical features

Overgrowth commences within the interdental papillae (Fig. 100) which enlarge until they coalesce, involving all of the attached gingiva (Fig. 101). Overgrowth extends coronally and may interfere with speech, occlusion and mastication. Aesthetics are severely compromised. Occasionally presents in the edentulous (Fig. 102).

Histopathology

Epithelium is parakeratinised and acanthotic, often with long, slender, elongated rete ridges. Fibrous tissue forms the bulk of the overgrowth, featuring a proliferation of fibroblasts and increased collagen content. Inflamed tissues are highly vascularised and contain collections of inflammatory cells. Plasma cells predominate, although lymphocytes and macrophages are also present.

Pathogenesis

The precise mechanism of overgrowth is uncertain and involves complex interactions between the drug, fibroblasts, plaque-induced inflammation and genetic factors. Sub-populations of fibroblasts exist which synthesise increased quantities of collagen, the relative proportions of which are genetically determined. Plaque-induced inflammation is a prerequisite for overgrowth and, in inflamed tissues, high-activity fibroblasts may become sensitised to the effects of systemic drugs. Human lymphocyte antigen (HLA) expression may be associated with fibroblast phenotype and could act as a marker for overgrowth.

Treatment

A strict programme of oral hygiene instruction and plaque control must be implemented. Overgrown tissues should be surgically excised.

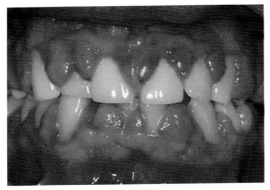

Fig. 100 Gingival overgrowth of interdental papillae.

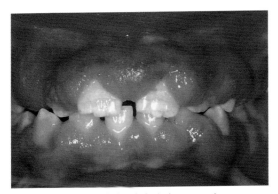

Fig. 101 Extensive drug-induced gingival overgrowth.

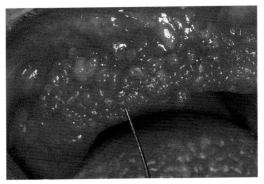

Fig. 102 Overgrowth in edentulous patient.

Crohn's disease

A chronic granulomatous disorder of unknown aetiology affecting any part of the gastrointestinal tract.

Clinical features

Oral manifestations include: oedema; hypertrophy and fissuring of the buccal mucosa ('cobblestone appearance'); swelling of the lips (Fig. 103) and cheeks; mucosal tags; oral ulceration; angular cheilitis. An erythematous granular enlargement of the entire width of the attached gingiva may be evident (Fig. 104).

Treatment

Oral hygiene instruction, scaling, root planing.

Orofacial granulomatosis (OFG)

Not a discrete clinical entity but describes the common clinicopathological presentation of a variety of disorders including Crohn's disease and some topical hypersensitivity reactions.

Acute leukaemia

A malignant proliferation of white blood cells and their precursors resulting in increased numbers of circulating leukocytes and infiltration of tissues by leukaemic cells. Periodontal manifestations include (Fig. 105):

- *gingival enlargement*; due to infiltration of the gingival connective tissues by leukaemic cells.
- *gingival bleeding*; results from thrombocytopenia which accompanies the leukaemia.
- *acute periodontal abscess*; develops from an acute exacerbation of pre-existing periodontitis.

Treatment

Oral hygiene is impaired by enlarged tissues. Chemical anti-plaque agents should be prescribed and acute infections managed with systemic antimicrobials.

(See pp. 129–130 for other haematological disorders.)

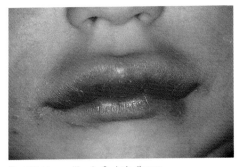

Fig. 103 Lip swelling in Crohn's disease.

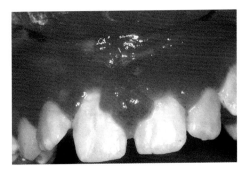

Fig. 104 Granulomatous gingival enlargement in Crohn's disease.

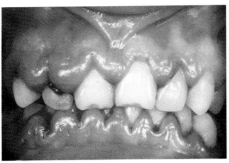

Fig. 105 Acute monocytic leukaemia—gingival swelling.

Sarcoidosis

A systemic chronic granulomatous disorder of unknown aetiology typically affecting the lungs, lymph nodes, liver, skin, and eyes.

Clinical features

Oral lesions are rare, but reported periodontal manifestations include a hyperplastic granulomatous gingivitis (Fig. 106). Altered lymphocyte and PMN function may (rarely) lead to rapid periodontal destruction.

Wegener's granulomatosis

A systemic disease characterised by necrotising granulomas of the respiratory system and kidneys, and necrotising vasculitis of small arteries.

Clinical features

A characteristic hyperplastic gingivitis with petechiae and an ulcerated 'strawberry' appearance (Fig. 107).

Treatment

Gingival condition improves when systemic drug therapy (prednisolone and cyclophosphamide) is initiated.

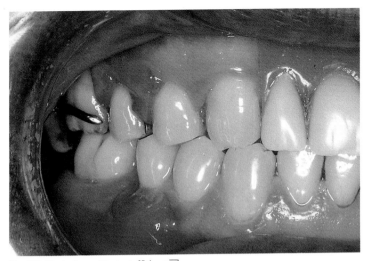

Fig. 106 Gingival sarcoidosis at $\underline{65}/$ and $\overline{57}$.

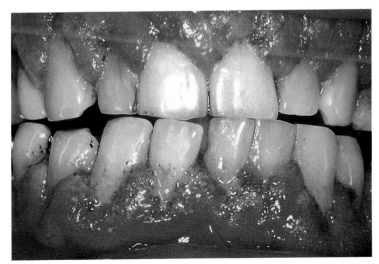

Fig. 107 Wegener's granulomatosis.

Epulides

Localised hyperplastic lesions arising from the gingiva.

Aetiology Trauma, and chronic irritation from plaque and calculus invoke a chronic inflammatory response in which continued inflammation and attempts at repair proceed concurrently. Excessive production of granulation tissue results, forming the epulis.

Clinical features *Fibrous epulis* (Fig. 108) A firm, pink, pedunculated mass which may be ulcerated if traumatised. Histologically, comprises chronically inflamed, hyperplastic fibrous tissue which may be richly cellular or densely collagenous. Metaplastic bone and/or foci of dystrophic calcification are common.

Vascular epulides   Pyogenic granuloma and *pregnancy epulis* (Fig. 109). A soft, purple-red swelling, frequently ulcerated, which bleeds readily. Histologically, a proliferation of richly vascular tissue supported by a fibrous stroma with a thin, often extensively ulcerated epithelium. A pregnancy epulis is a pyogenic granuloma occurring in a pregnant female. Vascular and fibrous epulides probably represent different phases of the same inflammatory process.

Peripheral giant cell granuloma (GCG) (Fig. 110)   A dark reddish purple, ulcerated swelling, frequently arising interdentally and often extending buccally and lingually. May cause superficial erosion of crestal alveolar bone. Radiographs are essential to differentiate from a central GCG which has perforated the cortex to present as a peripheral swelling. Histologically, contains multiple foci of osteoclast-like giant cells supported by a richly vascular and cellular stroma.

Treatment Surgical excision.
   Haemostasis may be problematic when removing pregnancy epulides. These can be left until after parturition as they then tend to reduce in size and become increasingly fibrous. Excision during pregnancy generally results in recurrence.

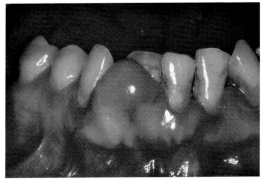

Fig. 108 Fibrous epulis.

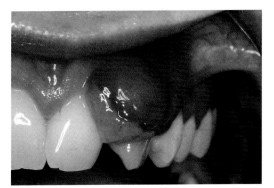

Fig. 109 Pregnancy epulis.

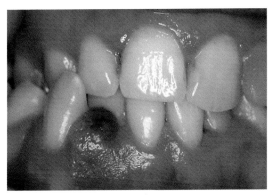

Fig. 110 Peripheral giant cell granuloma.

Iatrogenic enlargement

Denture induced
Chronic trauma from ill-fitting dentures can result in hyperplasia of the underlying gingival tissues (Fig. 111). Frequently associated with prostheses supported by mucosa only, with inadequate gingival clearance and poor stability.

Clinical features   Tissues may be oedematous but become increasingly fibrous in the long term.

Treatment   Oral hygiene instruction (OHI); denture hygiene; scaling and root planing; replacement of defective prostheses.

Orthodontically induced
Orthodontic movement of teeth occasionally results in the 'heaping-up' of gingival soft tissues in the direction of tooth movement. This occurs more frequently when teeth are repositioned with removable appliances (tipping movement) than with fixed appliances (bodily movement).

Clinical features   An accumulation of gingival soft tissues in the direction of tooth movement. Frequently affects the palatal gingiva adjacent to maxillary incisors when being retracted (Fig. 112). Tends to resolve on completion of orthodontic treatment.

Treatment   OHI; appliance hygiene.

Cystic lesions

Clinical features   *Gingival cysts* account for less than 1% of cysts of the jaws. They are more common in neonates, tending to resolve spontaneously in early life. In adults, they are generally chance findings in histological sections from gingivectomy specimens (Fig. 113). Typically asymptomatic. Probably odontogenic in origin, arising from remnants of the dental lamina.

Developmental lateral periodontal cyst   may present with expansion of alveolar bone, but most are incidental findings on radiographs. They resemble gingival cysts if arising near the alveolar bone crest. Radiographically, they appear as a radiolucency with well-defined bony margins.

Treatment   Surgical excision.

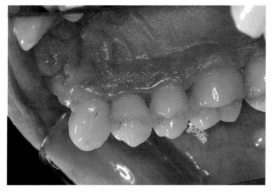

Fig. 111 Denture-induced overgrowth of free gingiva.

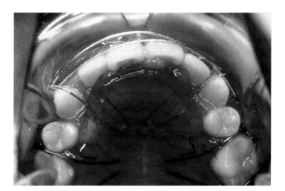

Fig. 112 Localised overgrowth palatal to retracted incisors.

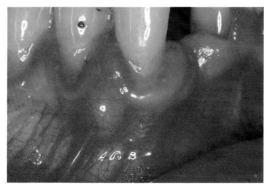

Fig. 113 Gingival cyst.

Gingival recession

Width of attached gingiva varies throughout the mouth (Fig. 114) and, in health, tends to increase with age. Labially, in both maxilla and mandible, the narrowest width is adjacent to the canines and premolars. The width may also be reduced considerably at sites adjacent to high frenal attachments. A band of attached gingiva is desirable to:

- maintain sulcus depth
- resist frictional forces from toothbrushing or mastication

When gingival recession occurs the width of attached gingiva is reduced or eliminated. A narrow, or finite width of attached gingiva is compatible with health (Fig. 115) and the width of attached gingiva alone should not be regarded as the only 'risk factor' for gingival recession. ➡

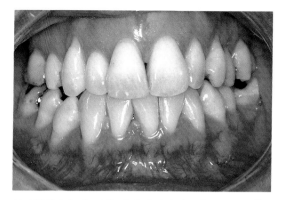

Fig. 114 Variation in width of attached gingiva. Compare maxilla with mandible.

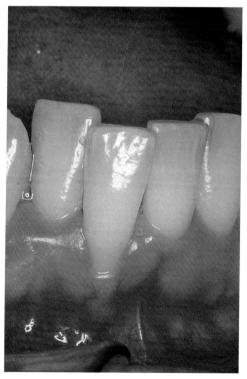

Fig. 115 Absence of attached gingiva labial to $\overline{1}$. Note healthy marginal tissue.

Gingival recession can affect any site in the mouth and, depending upon aetiological factors, may be localised or generalised.

Aetiology

There is often an element of trauma that can be identified as a contributing factor:

- Excessive toothbrushing force, incorrect technique or use of a particularly abrasive dentifrice (Fig. 116)
- Traumatic incisor relationships (Fig. 117)
- Habits such as rubbing the gingiva with a finger nail or the end of a pencil.

Recession is a consequence of periodontal disease (p. 27), periodontal treatment (Fig. 118) and a complication of orthodontic treatment when roots are moved labially through an existing dehiscence.

Complications

An exposed root surface on an anterior tooth is often aesthetically unacceptable. Exposure of dentine may cause extreme sensitivity and root surfaces are susceptible to caries. Sibilant speech may result from widened interdental spaces. ➡

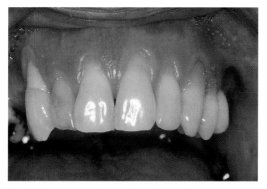

Fig. 116 Recession due to use of soot as dentifrice.

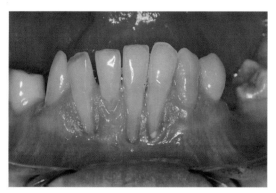

Fig. 117 Shearing of lower labial gingiva by maxillary incisors.

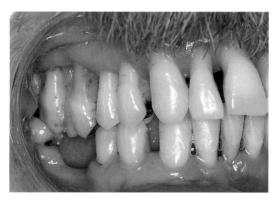

Fig. 118 Recession as a consequence of non-surgical periodontal treatment.

Apical migration of the gingival complex exposes the root surface. Wear cavities on root surfaces are indicative of toothbrush abrasion as an aetiological factor.

Stillman's cleft is an incipient lesion, a narrow, deep and slightly curved cleft extending apically from the free gingival margin (Fig. 119). As the recession progresses apically, the cleft becomes broader exposing the cementum of the root surface. When the lesion reaches the mucogingival junction the apical border of oral mucosa is usually inflamed because of the difficulty in maintaining good plaque control at this site (Fig. 120).

McCall's festoon is a rolled, thickened band of gingiva usually seen adjacent to canines when recession approaches the mucogingival junction (Fig. 121).

Dehiscences (clefts) or fenestrations (windows) are natural defects in labial alveolar plates which are often but not exclusively associated with prominent roots or teeth that are crowded out of the arch (Fig. 53). Such defects need not necessarily initiate recession but rather increase its rate of progression once established.

- Record the magnitude of recession.
- Eliminate aetiological factors.
- OHI.
- Topical desensitising agents/fluoride varnish.
- Gingival veneer to cover exposed roots/embrasure spaces.
- Surgical widening of attached gingiva if patient is unable to practice good oral hygiene because of local mucogingival morphology, or if recession progresses despite good plaque control.
- Crown teeth (after diagnostic wax up) but exercise extreme caution to prevent exposure of coronal pulp at level of radicular preparation.

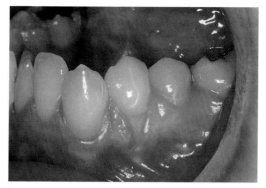

Fig. 119 Incipient Stillman's cleft.

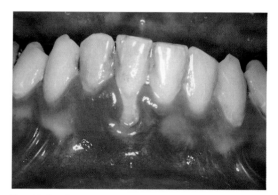

Fig. 120 Broad, deep gingival cleft with inflamed margins.

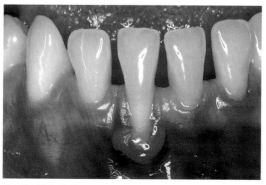

Fig. 121 McCall's festoon.

The periodontium has an inherent capacity to adapt to physiologic or traumatic forces that occur during normal or hyperfunction. In some cases the trauma exceeds the adaptive nature of the tissues and pathologic change and injury prevail.

Self-inflicted trauma

Factitious gingivitis

Minor form is seen in young children. Food packing or local inflammation provides a locus of irritation and the child picks or rubs the area with a finger nail (Figs 122, 123), pencil, or abrasive food such as crisps or nuts. If untreated, ulceration and inflammation persist and gingival recession may ensue. The lesion usually resolves when the habit is corrected. ➡

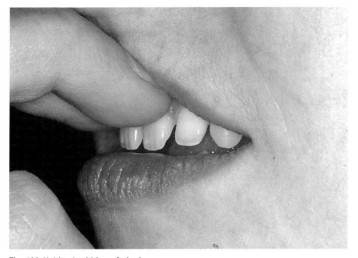

Fig. 122 Habitual rubbing of gingiva.

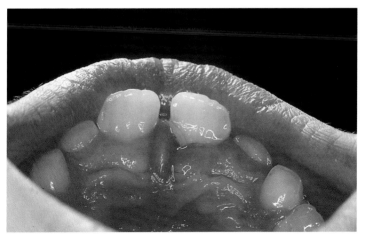

Fig. 123 Nail emerging from palatal of ⸤1⸥.

Major form lesions are more severe and widespread both intra- and extra-orally. They present as ulcers, abrasions, gingival recession, or blisters which may be blood-filled (Figs 124, 125, 126). Trauma may be inflicted subconsciously, or purposely in an attempt to deceive clinicians into diagnosing organic disease. The outlines of lesions provide clues as to the objects used to produce them. The lesions are remarkably resistant to conventional treatment and may reflect an underlying psychological problem. Referral to a psychologist/psychiatrist is advised but rarely welcomed by patients or relatives. ➡

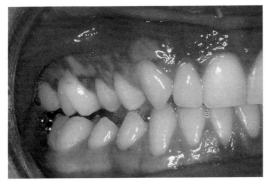

Fig. 124 Self-inflicted gingival ulceration.

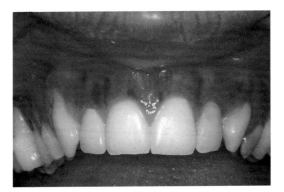

Fig. 125 Blood-filled blisters inflicted by finger nails.

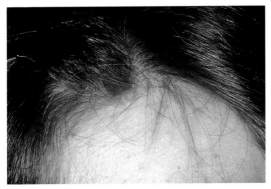

Fig. 126 Self-inflicted lesion on scalp.

Oral hygiene practices

Used incorrectly and without instruction, toothbrushes and interproximal cleaning aids can cause irreversible trauma to both periodontal tissues and teeth. Injudicious toothbrushing causes gingival abrasions, clefting and recession which can be localised or generalised (p. 91). Excessive toothbrushing force also produces typical V-shaped abrasion cavities. Localised defects can be caused by mini-interdental brushes, incorrect use of floss and dental woodpoints (Figs 127, 128, 129).

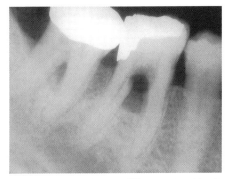

Fig. 127 Abrasion of furcation $\overline{6/}$ by interdental brush.

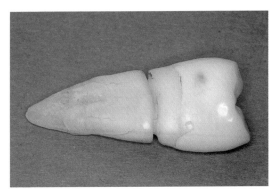

Fig. 128 Abraded root by habitual, excessive use of floss.

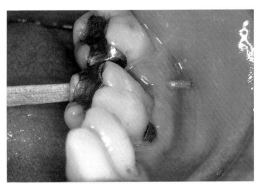

Fig. 129 Gingival perforation by incorrect use of woodstick.

Iatrogenic trauma

Dental procedures and components of poorly designed restorations or appliances can cause direct local irritation/trauma to the gingiva. Examples include:

- Injudicious use of rotary, ultrasonic, and scaling instruments (Fig. 130)
- Placement of excessive gingival retraction cord or leaving remnants of material in the gingival sulcus after taking an impression
- Spillage of caustic chemicals used in dental treatments (Fig. 131)
- Components of fixed/removable orthodontic appliances
- Components of removable partial dentures
- Extension of a palatal denture base into the interproximal areas to rest upon the gingival papillae (Fig. 132)

In the short term, traumatic lesions of the soft tissues are reversible when the stimulus is removed. More persistent, chronic irritation can lead to gingival recession.

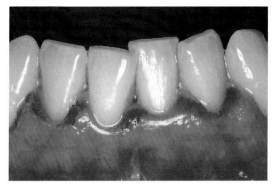

Fig. 130 Gingival abrasion caused by polishing brush.

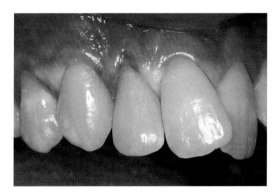

Fig. 131 Chemical burn with composite primer.

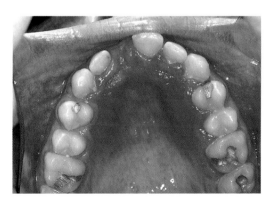

Fig. 132 Denture-induced stomatitis with trauma to marginal gingiva.

Jiggling forces

Forces acting successively, in opposite directions, thus preventing the tooth from moving orthodontically away from the forces, and subjecting the periodontium to alternating phases of pressure and tension. Such forces may originate from the components of removable prostheses or appliances.

Clinical features

In health there is an increase in tooth mobility until the periodontium adapts to the forces. Jiggling forces do not initiate attachment loss. In the presence of marginal periodontitis the rate of periodontal destruction increases and tooth mobility also increases progressively. The adaptive capacity of the periodontal ligament is reduced. Radiographically there is widening of the periodontal membrane space (Figs 133, 134).

Histopathology

Changes in the periodontal vasculature: proliferation of vessels, increased fluid exudation and thrombosis.

Treatment

Establish periodontal health and identify, then eliminate, the jiggling forces.

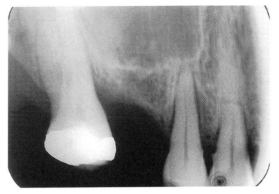

Fig. 133 Radiographic widening of periodontal membrane space on 5 / jiggled by denture.

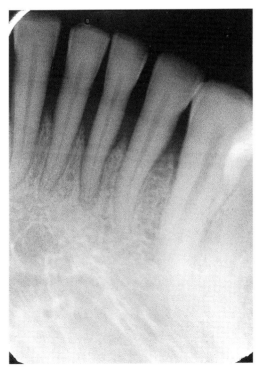

Fig. 134 /1 jiggled by bulky contour of upper crown (not shown).

Occlusal interferences

Occlusal interferences or premature occlusal contacts can arise when the occlusal morphology and/or position of teeth are altered, for example following placement of restorations or after orthodontic therapy.

Clinical features

Pain, fracture or faceting of cusps, attrition, bruxism, increased tooth mobility and temporomandibular joint symptoms. Radiographic widening of the periodontal membrane space suggests tissue remodelling as an attempt to adapt to the interference. Potentially, the most damaging interferences are due to premature contacts in retruded contact position or non-working contacts in lateral mandibular excursion. In the presence of periodontal inflammation a persistent interference with increased occlusal loading can produce localised, infrabony defects which may jeopardise the prognosis of the tooth (Figs 135, 136).

Treatment

Resolve periodontal inflammation. Identify clinically the interference. Confirm by mounting study models in retruded contact position on a semi-adjustable articulator. Occlusal adjustment.

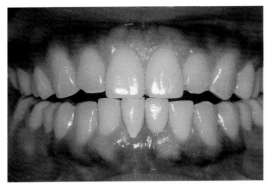

Fig. 135 Interference on $\overline{7|}$ in protrusion.

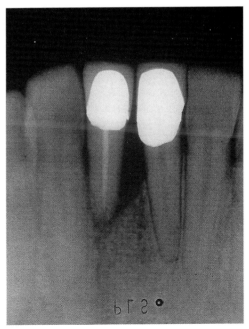

Fig. 136 Radiograph of $\overline{7|}$ showing extensive localised bone loss. Same patient as Fig. 135.

Traumatic incisor relationships

Classification

The Akerly classification identifies the relationship between the maxillary and mandibular incisors, and the nature of complete overbite.

Class I. Lower incisors impinge upon the palatal mucosa (Fig. 137).

Class II. Lower incisors occlude on the palatal gingival margins of the maxillary teeth (Fig. 138).

Class III. A deep, traumatic overbite (class II division 2) with shearing of the mandibular labial gingiva (Fig. 139).

Class IV. Lower incisors occlude with the palatal surfaces of upper incisors. Evidence of tooth wear due to attrition and minimal, if any, effect upon supporting tissues.

Aggravating factors

Inherent development of a severe, class II division 2 incisor relationship; injudicious orthodontic or restorative treatment; gradual loss of posterior support with distal movement of premolars and canines and the presence of powerful lip musculature.

Treatment

Interventive treatment of developmental cases in childhood. In adults, establish periodontal health, protect tissues temporarily with a soft acrylic splint, restore posterior dimension. More complex cases may require orthodontic therapy, orthognathic surgery, segmental or full mouth rehabilitation, with or without the use of Dahl and overlay appliances.

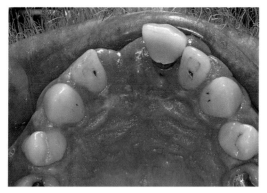

Fig. 137 Akerly class I. Note palatar imprints of lower incisors.

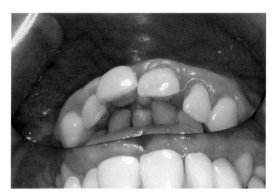

Fig. 138 Akerly class II.

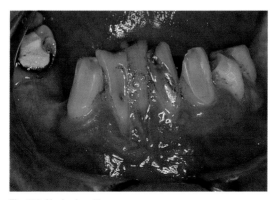

Fig. 139 Akerly class III.

Aggressive periodontal diseases which occur in apparently healthy individuals. They are characterised clinically by age of patient at onset and the extent and pattern of bone loss.

Prepubertal periodontitis (PP)

Clinical features

May be clinically detected as soon as the primary teeth erupt.

Generalised PP   Gingiva are fiery red, oedematous, swollen and haemorrhagic (Fig. 140). Gingival clefts and multiple sites of recession are evident. Bone loss is generalised and affects most teeth, which can be lost as early as 3–5 years of age (Fig. 141). Patients often suffer from general infections of the upper respiratory tract and middle ear.

Localised PP   Gingival changes and plaque deposits are minimal with only mild inflammation of the marginal tissues. Bone loss has a typical incisor–molar distribution, and the disease progression is slower than that of the generalised form.

Microbiology

A number of very aggressive periodontopathogens: *Actinobacillus actinomycetemcomitans, Porphyromonas gingivalis, Fusobacterium nucleatum, Eikenella corrodens*.

Investigations

There is some doubt whether PP is a phenotypically defined disease entity, or just one manifestation of underlying disease such as leukocyte adhesion deficiency (LAD) syndrome (p. 121). An exhaustive medical screen is thus indicated and long-term follow-up is essential.

Treatment

Localised PP usually responds well to conventional treatment: oral hygiene instruction, scaling and root planing. Antimicrobials indicated if infection persists and the disease is refractory to treatment. Extraction of teeth may help to restrict PP to the primary dentition.

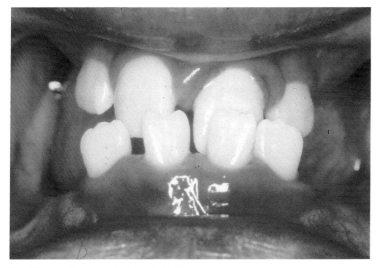

Fig. 140 Generalised prepubertal periodontitis.

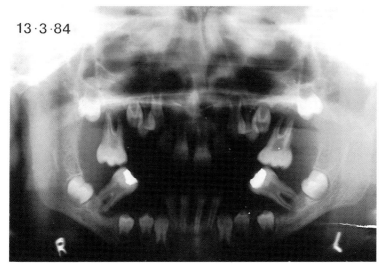

13·3·84

Fig. 141 Primary dentition lost. First molars and incisors affected at 7 years.

Juvenile periodontitis (JP)

Classically affects the permanent dentition with onset around puberty. Occasionally there may be a history of PP. Also presents in localised and generalised forms.

Epidemiology

Prevalence in developed countries is about 0.1%, but is somewhat higher in developing countries (0.5%). In the UK, prevalence is higher in certain ethnic groups: Asians (0.2%), Afro-Caribbeans (0.8%). There is no predilection for either sex.

Clinical features

Localised JP Characterised by pocketing, bleeding on probing, and loss of attachment (BPE 4) in the incisor–molar region. The gingiva can appear healthy (Fig. 142) when there are low levels of supragingival plaque. The radiographic pattern of bone loss is distinctive with bilateral angular defects around molars (Fig. 143) and horizontal loss around incisors. One or two premolars/canines may also be affected.

Generalised JP Pocketing is more widespread, affecting most if not all the teeth. Gingival bleeding can be profuse with a purulent exudate from deeper pockets. Periodontal abscesses may be the initial presenting sign.
  Bone loss is generalised and irregular with a combination of vertical and horizontal defects.
  The commonest presenting complaints of patients with JP are drifting of teeth and the appearance of spaces between the incisors (Fig. 144).

Microbiology

The subgingival flora comprises mainly Gram-negative, anaerobic periodontopathogens: *Actinobacillus actinomycetemcomitans, Capnocytophaga, Prevotella intermedia, Porphyromonas gingivalis, Eikenella corrodens.*

Pathology

Impaired neutrophil function with defects in both chemotaxis and phagocytosis. The defect in chemotaxis is believed to be transmitted as a dominant trait. There are also defects in cell-mediated immunity.

Treatment

Conventional treatment is frequently combined with systemic antimicrobial therapy: tetracycline, 250 mg q.d.s. for 2 weeks or a combination of metronidazole 400 mg + amoxycillin 500 mg b.d.

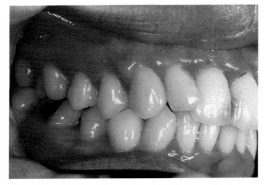

Fig. 142 Localised juvenile periodontitis with 'superficial' presentation of mild gingivitis.

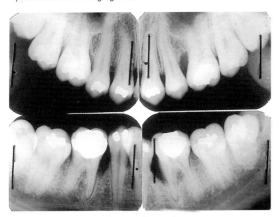

Fig. 143 Angular bone defects on first molars.

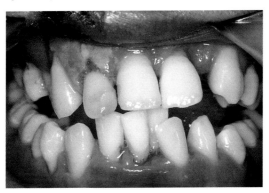

Fig. 144 Generalised juvenile periodontitis.

for 1 week. Ideally, however, the antimicrobial regimen should be based upon sampling pockets, culture and sensitivity testing. An antimicrobial regimen can also be used in conjunction with periodontal surgery. Long-term maintenance is essential. Family studies suggest that early onset diseases, and juvenile periodontitis in particular, are heritable traits with an autosomal recessive pattern. It is therefore important to screen siblings, and (eventually) offspring of affected individuals whenever possible.

Rapidly progressing adult periodontitis (RPP)

Clinical features

Age of onset is in early adulthood, between about 20 and 35 years of age (Figs 145, 146). The disease is usually generalised and characterised by marked gingival inflammation, pockets (BPE 4), bleeding (spontaneous, or after probing), and abscess formation. Bone resorption is very rapid and tooth loss is almost inevitable if the disease is untreated. In some instances the disease becomes quiescent or may convert to a more slowly progressing chronic adult periodontitis.

Microbiology and pathology

The subgingival flora is very similar to that of JP, and defects in leukocyte function have also been detected.

Differential diagnosis

Periodontitis associated with insulin-dependent diabetes.

Investigations

Enquire about family history of diabetes. Glucose tolerance test may reveal subclinical or early stages of juvenile diabetes.

Treatment

Extract teeth which have a hopeless prognosis. Conventional non-surgical management or surgical therapy to provide better access for root planing at sites of deep pockets. Systemic antimicrobial therapy (see JP) may also be indicated.

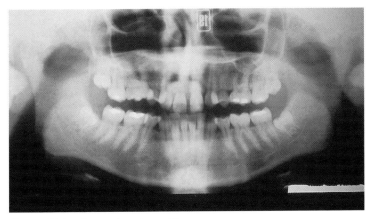

Fig. 145 Adult patient—no bone loss at 19 years.

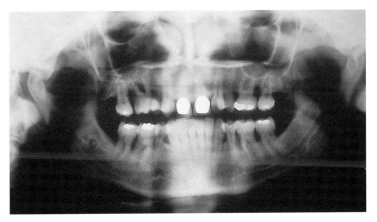

Fig. 146 Same patient with extensive bone loss at 34 years of age.

Early onset periodontal diseases (Ch. 15) are also a manifestation of several rare, but well-recognised heritable syndromes. Many of these syndromes are associated with profound abnormalities of neutrophil function which predispose these patients to their periodontal problems.

Papillon–Lefèvre syndrome

Incidence

A rare condition transmitted as an autosomal recessive trait with an estimated incidence of 1–4 per million births. A history of consanguinity between parents is found in about 30% of cases.

Clinical features

The syndrome is characterised by a diffuse palmar-plantar hyperkeratosis (Fig. 147) and a prepubertal periodontitis with onset at about 2 years of age. The child may be rendered edentulous by 5–6 years (Fig. 148). Progressive periodontal destruction usually also affects the permanent dentition with patients becoming edentulous by the age of 20. The clinical presentation may show wide variation; occasionally the skin and periodontal lesions present on their own as distinct clinical entities. Variations in periodontal presentation include cases which affect only the primary dentition, and a late onset disorder where the primary dentition remains unaffected.

Pathology

Defects in neutrophil adhesion, chemotaxis and phagocytosis have been observed in some patients.

Treatment

Intensive periodontal therapy includes oral hygiene instruction, chlorhexidine rinses, scaling, and prescription of antimicrobials (metronidazole and amoxycillin) to control acute phases. Severely involved teeth must be extracted. The loss of teeth is almost inevitable, even with a high degree of patient compliance. A more realistic aim is to maintain alveolar bone height to eventually support removable or implant-retained prostheses.

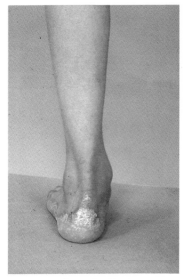

Fig. 147 Hyperkeratosis of heel.

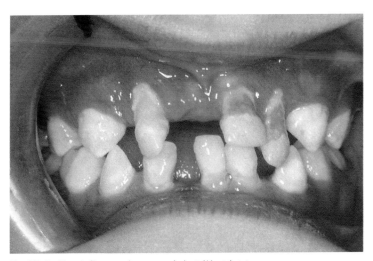

Fig. 148 Papillon–Lefèvre syndrome—periodontal/dental status.

Ehlers–Danlos syndrome

Transmitted as an autosomal dominant or recessive trait with the primary defect being with the synthesis and extracellular polymerisation of collagen molecules. Ten types have been described.

Clinical features

Excessive mobility of joints (Fig. 149) and increased extensibility of skin, which is also susceptible to bruising and scarring following superficial wounds. In types I and IV the oral soft tissues are prone to bruising and haemorrhage due to defective support of the lamina propria. Gingival bleeding may occur after toothbrushing. Patients with the type VIII variant appear especially susceptible to advanced periodontal disease (Fig. 150).

Pathology

Lesions are characterised by massive proliferation of Langerhans cells (resembling histiocytes) with varying numbers of eosinophils and multinucleate giant cells.

Histopathological changes of teeth have been detected: enamel hypoplasia, abnormalities of dentine and an increased incidence of pulp stones.

Treatment

Conventional treatment for periodontal disease but extreme caution must be taken because of the fragility of the soft tissues and their susceptibility to trauma.

Oral lesions are accessible for biopsy to confirm a diagnosis. Local excision and curettage of bone lesions is often successful although the prognosis is poor when soft tissues become widely involved. When a patient presents with oral lesions a complete radiographic screening or bone scan is needed to detect or exclude multifocal involvement.

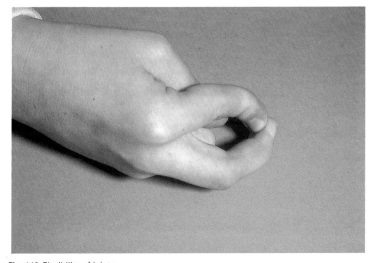

Fig. 149 Flexibility of joints.

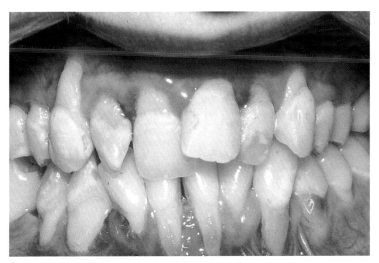

Fig. 150 Ehlers–Danlos syndrome—advanced periodontal disease.

Diabetes mellitus

A syndrome of metabolic disorders associated with an intolerance to glucose:

Type I—insulin-dependent diabetes mellitus; sudden onset predominantly in young adults

Type II—non-insulin-dependent; gradual onset in middle age.

General symptoms are thirst, hunger, polyuria and weight loss. The prevalence is about 2%.

Periodontal disease

Clinical features

Generally, the well-controlled diabetic is at no increased risk from periodontal disease. A poorly controlled diabetic with complications (nephropathy, retinopathy) is at risk from a rapidly progressing type of early onset periodontitis (Figs 151, 152). Multiple periodontal abscesses or suppurating pockets are a feature.

Aetiology

The subgingival microflora in diabetic patients contains recognised periodontopathogens: *Actinobacillus actinomycetemcomitans, Capnocytophaga, Prevotella intermedius, Campylobacter rectus, Porphyromonas gingivalis.* Several factors may contribute to the disease pathogenesis. Impaired neutrophil function includes reduced chemotaxis, phagocytosis and intracellular killing. Well-recognised vascular changes which accompany diabetes (thickening and hyalinisation of vascular walls) appear to have little, if any bearing on the periodontal status.

Treatment

Extraction of hopelessly involved teeth followed by conventional non-surgical or surgical therapy. Systemic antimicrobials (amoxycillin and metronidazole) are indicated for persistent or recurrent infections. In view of the susceptibility of diabetics to general infections antibiotic prophylaxis should be considered prior to periodontal surgery.

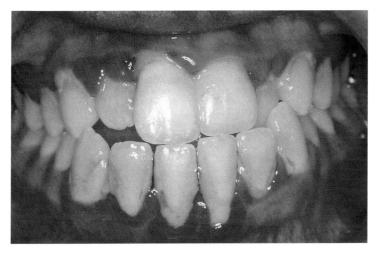

Fig. 151 Periodontal disease in type I diabetes.

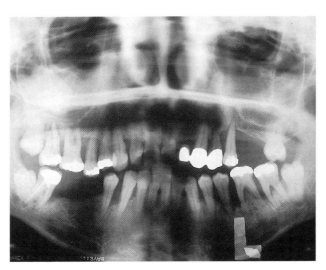

Fig. 152 Extensive bone loss in adult. Type II diabetes.

Leukocyte adhesion deficiency syndrome

A single gene defect with an autosomal recessive pattern of inheritance.

Clinical features

Delayed separation of the umbilical cord at birth. Impaired wound healing and severe, often life-threatening bacterial infections are characteristic. Prepubertal periodontitis is present with an acute gingivitis, profuse bleeding and suppurating pockets (Fig. 153). The permanent dentition is also affected. In mild variants, the disease appears stable over long periods, only for an acute phase to develop and the patient to deteriorate very rapidly. Usually fatal by about 30 years.

Pathology

Impaired adhesion of neutrophils to vessel walls due to restricted expression of cell surface integrins.

Treatment

Palliative treatment for periodontal disease, which is of secondary importance to the life-threatening infections which occur.

Langerhans cell histiocytosis (LCH)

A triad of conditions (previously known as histiocytosis X) characterised by focal or more widespread proliferation of histiocytic cells with features of Langerhans cells. The acute form, Letterer–Siwe disease, is usually fatal in infancy. Eosinophilic granuloma (unifocal) and Hand–Schüller–Christian disease (multifocal) are closely related.

Clinical features

Single or multiple osteolytic lesions can be generalised, involving the pituitary fossa and the frontal, orbital and sphenoid bones. Progressive involvement may cause diabetes insipidus and exophthalmos (Hand–Schüller–Christian syndrome). Osteolytic involvement of alveolar bone is more common in the mandible and presents as an early onset periodontitis with a generalised and irregular pattern of bone resorption. Involved bone shows radiolucencies of considerable size (Fig. 154). Pain and excessive tooth mobility are common early symptoms. Periodontal abscess formation is common and the gingiva can be swollen, oedematous, necrotic and ulcerated (Fig. 155).

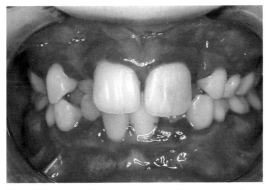

Fig. 153 Leukocyte adhesion deficiency syndrome—gingival condition.

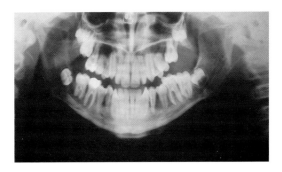

Fig. 154 Radiolucencies, predominantly of mandible, in LCH.

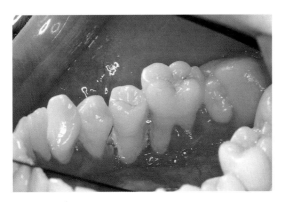

Fig. 155 Gingival ulceration and recession in LCH.

Down syndrome

Common autosomal chromosome abnormality—trisomy of number 21.

Incidence About 1:700 live births.

Clinical features Increased susceptibility to rapidly progressive or advanced type of periodontitis. Institutionalised patients have a greater prevalence of dental and periodontal problems than those cared for at home (Fig. 156). Local clinical factors which predispose to accumulation of dental plaque and restrict access for its removal include:
- class III malocclusion with crowding
- anterior open bite
- lack of lip seal leading to drying of plaque
- reduced salivary flow
- high frenal attachments
- tongue thrusting.

Treatment A good standard of plaque control is difficult to achieve due to lack of dexterity and motivation. Regular visits for scaling and prophylaxis.

Hypophosphatasia

An inborn error of metabolism with autosomal recessive and dominant patterns of inheritance. There is a deficiency of the liver/kidney/bone isoenzyme alkaline phosphatase which is crucial to the mineralisation of hard tissues.

Clinical features In juvenile (childhood) form bone defects can lead to mild bowing of the legs, proptosis and a delay in closure of the fontanelles. Aplastic or hypoplastic cementum leads to premature loss of the primary dentition (Fig. 157) due to extensive root resorption or bone loss as a result of a weakened periodontal attachment and disuse atrophy. The gingiva can appear quite healthy. In the adult form, which presents during middle age, the periodontal changes are localised to the incisor region.

Treatment When primary teeth are lost it is important to maintain space for their permanent successors which erupt prematurely.

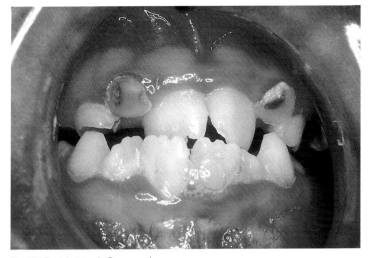

Fig. 156 Dental status in Down syndrome.

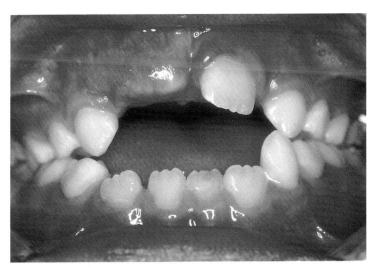

Fig. 157 Premature eruption of permanent teeth in a 4-year-old with hypophosphatasia.

The gingival lesions of mucocutaneous disorders may present as a non-specific, desquamative gingivitis (p. 21) but can also show more characteristic lesions similar to those seen elsewhere on the oral mucosa.

Lichen planus

A disease of unknown aetiology which is more prevalent in middle-aged females. Oral and gingival lesions appear in approximately 70% and 20% of cases respectively.

Gingival lesions

The presentation is variable but gingival lesions can appear as:
- white keratotic lesions (Fig. 158) which may be papular, linear, or resemble the characteristic lacy network of Wickham's striae
- vesiculobullous lesions
- large erosive patches or ulcers (Fig. 159)
- generalised atrophy and desquamation

Oral lichenoid reactions can be induced by systemic or local factors including drugs (chlorpropamide, methyldopa, gold salts, propanolol) and dental amalgam (Fig. 160).

Treatment

Reassurance and maintenance of a high standard of oral hygiene. During the acute, painful stage use chlorhexidine gluconate rinses for plaque control. Topical steroids: hydrocortisone hemisuccinate pellets (2.5 mg) held against the lesions 3 times a day or Becotide spray.

Long-term follow-up monitoring of ulcerative/atrophic forms is advisable as there is some evidence to suggest that these lesions may be slightly more at risk of malignant change.

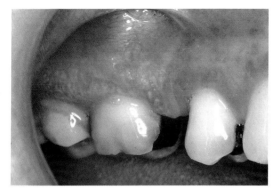

Fig. 158 White keratotic gingival lesion in lichen planus.

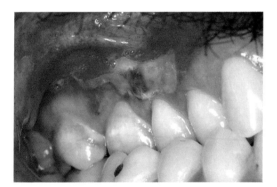

Fig. 159 Erosive lichen planus.

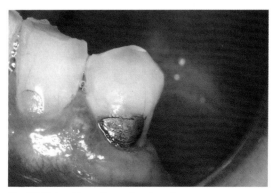

Fig. 160 Lichenoid reaction to dental amalgam.

Benign mucous membrane pemphigoid (BMMP)

An autoimmune, vesiculobullous condition which is more common in females and has an onset in middle age.

Clinical features

In addition to the oral mucosa, lesions can affect nasal, oesophageal and rectal mucosa. The most problematic lesions are those affecting the eyes causing conjunctivitis and, in severe cases, blindness. Intra-orally, fluid- or blood-filled vesicles (Fig. 161) affect the attached gingiva. Vesicles rupture after a short time leaving ulcers which heal without scarring. Epithelium is fragile and more generalised involvement appears as a desquamative gingivitis.

Treatment

Topical steroids. Sulcular toothbrushing technique to minimise gingival contact, and chemical plaque control during the acute phase. Regular observation of patients in the long term to check for development of eye lesions.

Pemphigus vulgaris

Rare, autoimmune, vesiculobullous disease affecting older patients and particularly those of Mediterranean origin.

Clinical features

Lesions affect the skin as well as the mucosa of eyes, nose, genitalia and larynx. Fluid-filled bullae which rupture, ulcerate and heal without scarring affect attached gingiva (Fig. 162) and other intra-oral sites. Painful oral lesions inhibit good plaque control, and are often the presenting sign of the disease. The bullae/vesicles may be present against a background of desquamative gingivitis.

Diagnosis

Nikolsky sign. Gentle rubbing of the gingiva causes stripping of the epithelium from the surface. This sign can also be elicited in pemphigoid so a biopsy is required to confirm the diagnosis.

Treatment

Topical corticosteroids for oral lesions. Sulcular toothbrushing technique using a soft brush to minimise trauma to gingiva. Chemical plaque control (chlorhexidine gluconate rinses) when brushing becomes too painful.

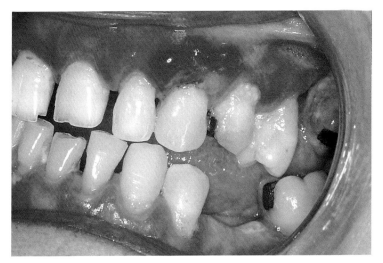

Fig. 161 Blood-filled vesicles on gingiva in BMMP.

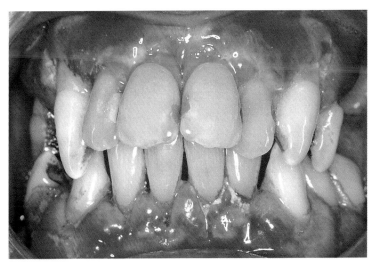

Fig. 162 Generalised gingival ulceration in pemphigus vulgaris.

Neutropenia

Benign familial, severe familial and cyclic neutropenia are heritable blood disorders which are characterised by a periodic (3-weekly) or prolonged fall in circulating neutrophils. The conditions are transmitted as autosomal dominant traits.

Clinical features

Patients are susceptible to recurrent or persistent oral and more generalised skin infections, the severity of which is usually associated with the degree of neutropenia. Periodontal manifestations of the different neutropenias can be very similar. Gingivae are bright, fiery red, oedematous and swollen, and bleed readily on probing (Fig. 163). Areas of gingival recession are often evident. Alveolar bone loss is either generalised or has the very characteristic incisor–molar pattern of localised prepubertal or juvenile periodontitis. Recurrent oral ulceration is a problem.

Treatment

Supportive therapy with a strict oral hygiene programme. Chemical plaque control with antimicrobial mouthrinses when oral ulceration restricts mechanical plaque control. Systemic antimicrobials are indicated during acute phases of periodontal infection with multiple abscess formation.

Aplastic anaemia

Clinical features

Compromised haemopoiesis with fatty replacement of the bone marrow and pancytopenia: anaemia, neutropenia, thrombocytopenia. The condition is induced by radiation, chemicals, drugs, infection and neoplasia. Bleeding associated with gingivitis is profuse (Fig. 164) and persistent because of the reduction in platelets.

Treatment

Conventional periodontal management. Liaise with medical practitioner and haematologist regarding the need for antibiotic cover and platelet transfusion.

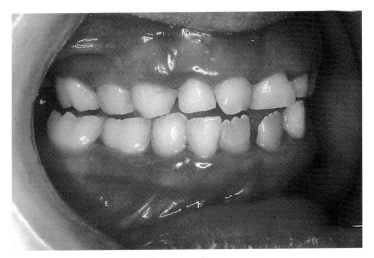

Fig. 163 Gingival appearance in cyclic neutropenia.

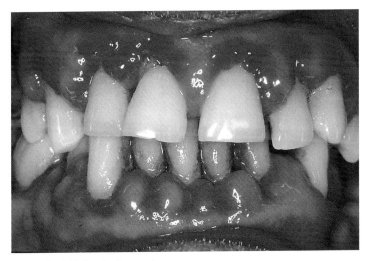

Fig. 164 Gingivitis in aplastic anaemia.

Haemangioma

Clinical features

Primarily affects the tongue, lips, cheeks and palate, though localised (Fig. 165) and generalised (Fig. 166) gingival lesions are also reported. Lesions are flat or raised, deep red-purple in colour, soft, and typically blanch under pressure. They may involve bone, muscle, salivary glands and present extra-orally. Lesions are generally considered to be hamartomatous in origin, not truly neoplastic.

Treatment

Radiography (including angiography) to determine full extent. Surgical excision, cryotherapy, sclerosing agents if appropriate. Dental procedures undertaken in the vicinity of an untreated lesion must proceed with care to prevent haemorrhage. Severe (occasionally uncontrollable) bleeding may result from unwary surgical treatment, including extractions.

Squamous cell papilloma

Clinical features

Benign tumour of oral mucosa, presenting on gingiva (Fig. 167), cheeks, lips, tongue, palate. Warty appearance with a white or pink surface depending on the quantity of keratin present. The precise aetiology is unclear, though human papilloma virus (HPV) has been implicated. HPV is also associated with *viral warts*, which may affect the oral mucosa, including the common wart (verruca vulgaris) and the venereal wart (condyloma acuminatum).

Treatment

Surgical excision.

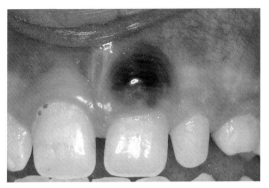

Fig. 165 Localised gingival haemangioma.

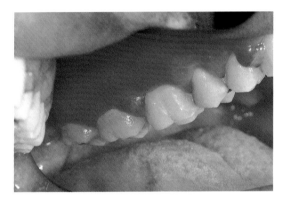

Fig. 166 Generalised gingival haemangioma.

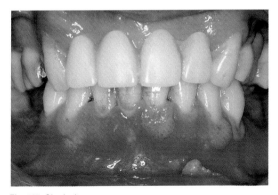

Fig. 167 Gingival warts.

Squamous cell carcinoma (SCC)

Incidence

Accounts for approximately 90% of oral malignancies, which in turn comprise 1–4% of all malignancies (UK). Traditionally a disease of the elderly (>50 years) and of men, though there is a trend towards equality between the sexes and presentation in younger age groups. There are approximately 2000 new cases per year and 1000 deaths (UK). Affects any part of the oral mucosa, including lip, tongue, floor of mouth, buccal mucosa and gingiva (Fig. 168).

Clinical features

Early presentation: white patch, small painless ulcer, exophytic growth, erythroplakia. *Late presentation*: (Fig. 168) hard persistent indurated ulcer with rolled edges; fixation to underlying tissues; pain; bleeding; alveolar bone destruction; regional lymph node involvement (reactive hyperplasia or metastatic spread).

Treatment

Surgical excision and reconstruction; radiotherapy; long-term follow-up.

Malignant melanoma

Clinical features

Rarely affects the oral mucosa, though very occasionally develops in the gingival tissues (Fig. 169). Presents as a dark brown or black lesion which tends to grow rapidly, invade bone and metastasise early. Prognosis is usually poor due to late presentation and the aggressive nature of the disease.

Treatment

Radical surgical excision and reconstruction; long-term follow-up.

Kaposi's sarcoma

Clinical features

The gingiva is a common site for the development of Kaposi's sarcoma in HIV-positive patients (Fig. 170). The lesion, of vascular origin, presents as a red or blue diffuse enlargement of a papilla before becoming generalised, invading alveolar bone and causing increased tooth mobility.

Treatment

Surgical excision, radiotherapy, chemotherapy.

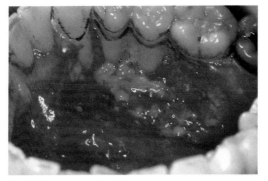

Fig. 168 Squamous cell carcinoma.

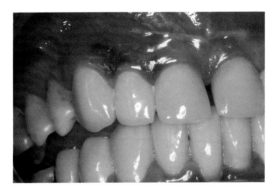

Fig. 169 Malignant melanoma of gingiva.

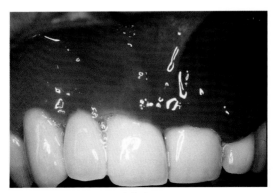

Fig. 170 Kaposi's sarcoma of gingiva.

An inflammatory condition of the tissues surrounding a functioning implant, with associated loss of supporting bone. (Distinguished from 'peri-implant mucositis' which is a reversible inflammatory reaction in the soft tissues.) The incidence appears to be 5–10%.

Aetiology

Plaque-associated inflammation is the main cause, but unfavourable occlusal loading must be considered where bone loss is evident (Fig. 171). The movement and loading of mobile mucosa overlying exposed implant screwthreads may be contributory, and the exposure of threads or rough implant surfaces in the mouth predispose to plaque accumulation. Microbiota from within the implant system cause inflammation at submucosal junctions, especially with loose abutments (Fig. 172). Trauma from brushing or food may provoke the condition. Drug-induced peri-implant mucosal overgrowth has also been reported.

Clinical features

Soreness, swelling, granulation tissue, bleeding and suppuration are invariably present (Fig. 172) with associated lymphadenopathy. Swollen tissue may prevent access for cleaning. Fistulae may be present in more chronic cases. Affected implant sites are often surrounded by mobile parakeratinised mucosa with little or no adjacent sulci. Bleeding on probing is seen in both conditions but probing attachment loss indicates peri-implantitis (Fig. 173).

Radiographic features

OPG or, ideally, long-cone periapical views reveal vertical or horizontal bone loss (Fig. 171), poor bony apposition and any inadequate seating of abutments or prosthesis/crown.

Management

Early detection by regular probing and radio-graphs. Improved plaque control and professional cleaning with or without topical antimicrobials usually suffices for the milder conditions. Cases with significant bone loss may require systemic antimicrobials and/or surgical repair, including guided bone regeneration (Fig. 171).

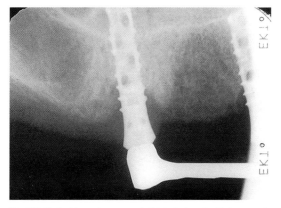

Fig. 171 Vertical bone loss around distal abutment with increased probing depth.

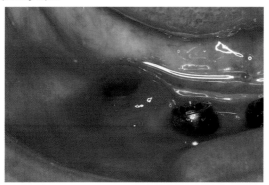

Fig. 172 Granulation tissue covers a loose abutment and prevents access for cleaning.

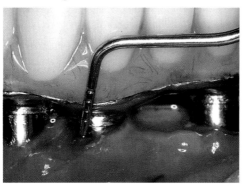

Fig. 173 Bleeding and increased probing attachment level in mobile mucosa. Note no sulcus.

Index